T0208986

9-Day Liver Detox Success Stories

How I felt before: I was very tired and lacking in energy. My sleep was not refreshing, and I often woke up feeling as though I hadn't had any sleep at all. I felt bloated and had achy joints.

How I felt after: My energy levels are much improved. I feel more refreshed in the morning; consequently, I feel more alert. The bloatedness has gone too, and, while I didn't do the program to lose weight, I've lost three pounds.

—Sophia Rauf

How I felt before: I felt tired, reliant on coffee to get going in morning, sluggish digestion, always bloated, sugar highs and lows, and craved pick-me-up snacks, like sweets, chocolate, or a coffee drink.

How I felt after: My body felt so good, the only thing I've reintroduced today (Day 10) is one small cup of tea. I have so much more energy, and getting up in the morning is far less painful. Digestion feels better and bowel movements are daily as opposed to twice weekly or even weekly!

—Jo Tongue

How I felt before: I felt lethargic and sluggish. I was always tired and always had a very bloated tummy. Every day I had painful arthritis in my neck and so took between three and five pain medications a day.

How I felt after: I have tons more energy. My work colleagues said they've noticed a difference in my skin and the way I move around with more energy and enthusiasm. After a couple of days, I no longer needed to take any pain medication. I have also lost four pounds, which seems to have gone from my waist area. I am very pleased with my improved appearance. I feel like a different person and would recommend it to everyone.

—Sandra Murray

How I felt before: I felt bloated, and lacked energy and interest in most things. I had poor concentration and was generally lethargic. I would start something but would not be able to finish anything.

How I felt after: I feel happier within myself. My energy levels are much higher: I look forward to taking on new tasks and am able to complete outstanding projects. At work, there seem to be fewer stressful situations. My skin looks healthier, and the dark circles under my eyes have improved.

—Margaret Davidson

Also by Patrick Holford

The Optimum Nutrition Bible

The 10 Secrets of 100% Healthy People

Food Glorious Food
(with Fiona McDonald Joyce)

How to Quit Without Feeling S**t
(with David Miller, PhD, and Dr. James Braly)

The Holford Low-GL Diet Cookbook
(with Fiona McDonald Joyce)

Smart Food for Smart Kids
(with Fiona McDonald Joyce)

The Low-GL Diet Bible

Patrick Holford's New Optimum Nutrition for the Mind

Optimum Nutrition for Your Child
(with Deborah Colson)

Food Is Better Medicine Than Drugs
(with Jerome Burne)

500 Health and Nutrition Questions Answered

Hidden Food Allergies
(with Dr. James Braly)

Optimum Nutrition Before, During and After Pregnancy
(with Susannah Lawson)

THE 9-DAY LIVER DETOX DIET

THE 9-DAY
LIVER
DETOX
DIET

The Definitive Diet
That Delivers Results

PATRICK HOLFORD *and*
FIONA MCDONALD JOYCE

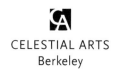

CELESTIAL ARTS
Berkeley

The information contained in this book is based on the experience and research of the author. It is not intended as a substitute for consulting with your physician or other health care provider. Any attempt to diagnose and treat an illness should be done under the direction of a health care professional. The publisher and author are not responsible for any adverse effects or consequences resulting from the use of any of the suggestions, preparations, or procedures discussed in this book.

First published in Great Britain in 2007 by Piatkus Books, an imprint of Little, Brown Book Group

Library of Congress Cataloging-in-Publication Data
Holford, Patrick.
  The 9-day liver detox diet : the definitive diet that delivers results / Patrick Holford, Fiona McDonald Joyce.
     p. cm.
Includes bibliographical references and index.
1. Liver—Popular works. 2. Diet therapy—Popular works.
3. Detoxification (Health) I. McDonald Joyce, Fiona. II. Title.
III. Title: Nine-day liver detox diet.
RC846.H65 2010
616.3'620654—dc22
                                    2010045599

ISBN: 978-1-58761-037-0

Design by Chloe Rawlins

First Edition

147028534

Acknowledgments

I would especially like to thank my wonderful coauthor, Fiona, who is not only a great cook and nutritionist, but super efficient! Also Rachel Nicoll and Virginia Harry for their help researching for this book, and Jo Brooks and Jan Cutler at Piatkus Books for their tireless editing. Most of all, thanks to my wife, Gaby, for her help and encouragement and for working around the clock, and to all the willing volunteers who tried and tested the 9-Day Liver Detox Diet.

Contents

PART ONE

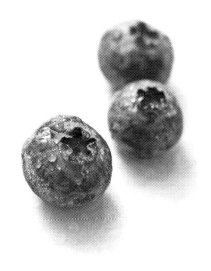

Introduction

Thirty years ago, I was introduced to the concept that most common Western diseases were largely the result of less-than-perfect nutrition. Although I was skeptical to begin with, after two months on a diet packed with fresh fruit and vegetables and supported by nutritional supplements, I saw the evidence for myself: I looked well, felt great, and had more vitality and mental clarity than ever before.

This experience was the beginning of a lifelong journey that resulted in my founding the Institute for Optimum Nutrition (ION) in 1984, with the help and support of two-time Nobel laureate Dr. Linus Pauling. ION, an independent nonprofit educational charity, is now one of the leading schools in Europe for training nutritional therapists. Its purpose is to educate the public and health professionals about the importance of optimum nutrition through its own publications, educational courses, and community outreach programs. ION also advises people on nutritional therapy and offers treatment where necessary.

Over the years, I have traveled all over the world lecturing on nutrition, as well as writing twenty-two books explaining how the food we eat and the liquids we drink have a direct effect on our health. During that time, it has been an honor to work with many great pioneers of what Linus Pauling called orthomolecular medicine, which simply translates as "giving the body the right molecules." He believed that optimum nutrition is the medicine of tomorrow, and he was right.

Since the foundation of ION, great advances have been made, with new research being published almost daily, proving the inextricable linking of health, disease, and nutrition. What those of us at the cutting edge of this new science have proven, day after day, in our clinics and with our research, is now finally being heralded by many as "the truth," as an abundance of research studies report on the restorative power of nutrients. For many years, nutritional therapists have been treating people who are unwell—whether vertically ill (upright but not feeling great) or horizontally ill (debilitated). These people have often consulted the therapists as a last resort, and we have seen clients restored to health and well-being beyond their wildest dreams.

You, too, can have optimum health—and there's no better way to kick-start it than with my 9-Day Liver Detox! Many of us recognize that some foods and drinks instantly make us feel good, and we may also know that there are other foods whose beneficial effects we feel the day after—perhaps making us feel more energized or refreshed. So we may already have an idea of what good nutrition does for us. Although many people have the mistaken idea that nutritionists are born virtuous and healthy, the truth is that most of us, just like you, have discovered optimum nutrition as the only sustainable solution for our own health problems or to create the feeling of well-being.

Why a liver detox?

This detox program concentrates on the liver, so you may be wondering why the liver is such an important organ in the body. In fact, the liver is the greatest multitasking organ, and as a result its function—or dysfunction—has an incredibly important impact on our health. Following are the liver's main functions.

Breaking down and eliminating toxins. The liver is the organ of detoxification. When it is not working properly, toxins from both inside and outside the body remain in the system and can cause your immune system to treat them as if they were invading organisms. This can lead to many health problems, including inflammation, increased likelihood of infections, and food allergies and sensitivities.

Breaking down and eliminating excess hormones. When this function is not working optimally, all kinds of hormonal imbalances can occur, promoting health problems from premenstrual syndrome (PMS) to acne.

Balancing blood sugar. When our blood sugar levels are high (for example, just after consuming sugary foods and drinks), the hormone insulin triggers the liver to store the excess as glycogen. When blood sugar levels fall, the liver releases glycogen to be turned into glucose. If the liver fails in this task, the result is chronic fatigue, sugar cravings, weight gain, and, ultimately, diabetes.

Producing bile. This vital substance helps digestion by breaking down fat and removing excess cholesterol. Without it, cholesterol levels rise and many digestive disorders can result, including bloating, irritable bowel syndrome (IBS), nausea, food allergies, and the malabsorption of nutrients, especially the fat-soluble vitamins A, D, E, and K.

Storing nutrients. The liver stores many essential vitamins and minerals, including iron, copper, and vitamins A, B12, D, E, and K.

In fact, just about any allergic, inflammatory, or metabolic disorder may involve or create impaired liver function, increasing inflammation in the body and resulting in eczema, asthma, chronic fatigue, chronic infections, inflammatory bowel disorders, multiple sclerosis, and rheumatoid arthritis, to name but a few, which in turn affect liver function.

Because the liver struggles valiantly on, working hard, it can be some time before serious symptoms of dysfunction appear. However, you may find that you are feeling tired and sluggish—this is a possible sign that your liver may benefit from a detox. You can check whether a detox would be beneficial for you by completing my questionnaire on page 12.

Are liver detoxes safe?

In the old days of total fasts, where you drank only water, naturopaths used to talk about the "healing crisis," when you felt worse before you felt better. But often this was really just a crisis! For safety, our bodies store toxins in our adipose tissue (fat stores). When we lose weight rapidly, those toxins are released, and the liver—as an organ of detoxification—has to deal with them. The idea of a liver detox is to support and take the load off the organ by providing the nutrients it needs—not to give it even more work to do!

My 9-Day Liver Detox is built on nothing but sound nutritional principles. It aims to support your liver's ability to do its job detoxing your body by removing antinutrients—in other words, toxins—from the diet and replacing them with the very nutrients it needs for optimum efficiency. You will not be starving yourself at any point; our 9-Day Menu Plan is carefully crafted, consisting of tasty, nutritious, and filling recipes so that you will never go hungry. Instead, you will be taking in a large quantity of the nutrients that are directly beneficial to your liver and which will actively support its detoxification function. It can then do its job of safely removing toxins from your fat stores and processing them appropriately without any ill effects.

Of course, if you are addicted to caffeine and go cold turkey while you follow the detox, you may feel worse for a couple of days, but soon you'll have more energy than ever before. You may get temporary withdrawal symptoms when you stop eating foods that you are intolerant to, but taking the recommended supplements really helps to minimize them. What you will be including in your diet will support not only your liver but the rest of your body, including your brain.

What benefits will you experience?

If you follow the steps in my 9-Day Liver Detox carefully, you should enjoy:

* Increased energy and vitality
* Clearer skin
* Freedom from digestive complaints
* Regular bowel movements
* Fresh breath
* Clearer sinuses
* Fewer infections
* Brighter eyes
* A sharper mind

You may even want to stay on the plan longer, for even more noticeable benefits.

Practicing what we preach

Fiona McDonald Joyce, who has provided all the wonderful recipes for this book, is a qualified ION nutritional therapist and cooking consultant. Her specialty is making what's good for you taste great. In advance of her wedding and while she was devising these recipes, she followed my 9-Day Liver Detox herself to solve some skin problems. She is happy to report great results—she looked absolutely radiant on her wedding day!

I am passionate about the healing power of my 9-Day Liver Detox, and it was exactly what I needed recently, having just completed a grueling lecture tour abroad, followed by a house move combined with some overindulgence over Easter. Within just two days, I felt completely recharged and back to tip-top health. It's amazing how good you can feel in such a short space of time.

Throughout this book, you will read many more firsthand experiences of what it is like to cut out favorite foods and the importance of having appetizing recipes when you are craving "off-limits" foods. You'll discover many recipes that are appetizing, interesting, and positively packed with nutrients that will become staples in your repertoire long after the nine days, making my 9-Day Liver Detox a highly doable and enjoyable experience.

The detox program will give you foods that boost your liver's ability to detoxify, plus liver-friendly supplements, so that you will start to feel better almost immediately. One skeptical journalist, Zoe Strimpel from the *Daily Telegraph*, "test-drove" the detox only, without the supplements, for just one day and said, "I must admit, I felt clearheaded and wholesome."

Let's face it—change is difficult. But the fear is usually of leaving the known—of breaking your unconscious food habits and doing something different. Once you start eating new foods that taste great and fill you up, it is remarkably easy. Here's how the book is arranged:

* Chapters 1, 2, and 3 explain exactly how your liver detoxifies, the five habits to break and the five habits to make, and the reasons behind them, to make your detox successful.

* Chapter 4, Test Your Detox Potential—Before and After, helps you identify, and quantify, your need to detox, with both questionnaires and a simple urine test that measures your detox potential.

* Chapter 5, Start Detoxing Now! tells you exactly what you need to do.

* Chapter 6, Your 9-Day Liver Detox Recipes, gives you exact daily menus and recipes so that you can follow the detox to the letter if you wish, or adapt it as you like according to your tastes.

* Chapter 7, Your Liver Detox for Life, explains how to reintroduce foods after the nine-day program, and how to learn what suits you in the process, and then to incorporate my detox principles into your daily life.

Overall, I expect you to enjoy the experience and love the results when you reach the end. It does take courage and commitment to say no to prepared foods and to the millions of other temptations, even for a week, but as you progress on the detox you will feel so many benefits that they will spur you on to continue. I wish you well, and as the old Chinese proverb says, "Perseverance furthers."

Chapter One

Why Detox?

Some people say that all you need to do to detox your body is to drink water and cut back on alcohol, so is detoxifying a myth and detox diets just a fad? In this chapter I will explain how toxins can build up in your body and create health problems, and how detoxing using supplements to assist the process can return you to a feeling of good health.

In this book, you will learn that your body expends as much effort detoxifying toxins as it does building new cells, but that your ability to detoxify is finite. Each of us is unique, both in which toxins we react to and in our ability to clear them from our body. When your body is detoxifying efficiently, the immediate effect is that you feel better, but efficient detoxification also has the potential to extend your healthy life, so understanding how detoxification works is an essential step toward improving your overall health. There are two sides to detoxifying: the first is to reduce the toxins your body is exposed to, and the second is to improve your body's ability to detoxify. There are three main areas in your body where this takes place: your digestive tract, your liver, and your immune system—and this means that your whole body is involved in the process.

My 9-Day Liver Detox is not like one of the trendy detox diets that you may have tried or read about. All of its principles are based on scientific fact (and for those who want to check them, I've not only listed all the references to the studies in the book but you can also visit www.patrickholford.com to find new information as it is published). This is science—not science fiction.

The reason why detox diets are so popular is that many people—probably including yourself—are well aware that they feel under par after a period of excess; this might be after too much sugar, caffeine, alcohol, fried food, overeating, active or secondhand smoke, exposure to pollution, or drugs. But you may also feel that your body has been affected by certain environments—perhaps moldy places or places that involve chemical exposure, for example—or after you have eaten certain foods. These are all examples of substances the body has to work hard to detoxify. Exactly how the body does this is the key to understanding how to boost your detox potential and feel better faster.

Our health now

Most of us are "vertically ill"—that is, we are upright but don't feel great. In this state, the balance between our intake of toxins and our ability to detoxify is not at its best. Some of us become "horizontally ill" and keel over when our intake of toxins exceeds our body's capacity to detoxify. Excess alcohol is an example of such a situation. When the liver's capacity to detoxify the alcohol you are consuming is exceeded, your brain becomes intoxicated and you become unable to stay conscious. Another example is the painkiller acetaminophen. When your liver is unable to detoxify that drug any longer, you'll collapse, and provided you make it to the hospital in time, you'll be pumped full of a detoxifying nutrient called glutathione to increase your liver's detoxing potential—and your liver will be back on track. Many old people die when their liver's ever-decreasing ability to detoxify is overloaded.

Right now, you are probably somewhere between the extremes of optimal and minimal detox potential. If you have the time and money, you can actually test your liver's ability to detoxify (more on this in chapter 4). For now, though, you can get an instant impression of your detox potential by completing the questionnaire below, which lists the symptoms associated with a reduced detox potential. Score yourself now and then retake the questionnaire and compare the score after completing my 9-Day Liver Detox.

QUESTIONNAIRE check your detox potential
Complete this questionnaire to discover whether you need to improve your detoxification potential:

1. Do you often suffer from headaches or migraine? ❑

2. Do you sometimes have watery or itchy eyes, or swollen, red, or sticky eyelids? ❑

3. Do you have dark circles under your eyes? ❑

4. Do you sometimes have itchy ears, earache, ear infections, drainage from the ears, or ringing in the ears? ❑

5. Do you often suffer from excessive mucus, a stuffy nose, or sinus problems? ❑

6. Do you suffer from acne, skin rashes, or hives? ❑

7. Do you sweat a lot and have a strong body odor? ❑

8. Do you sometimes have joint or muscle aches or pains? ❑

9. Do you have a sluggish metabolism and find it hard to lose weight, or are you underweight and find it hard to gain weight? ❑

10. Do you often suffer from frequent or urgent urination? ❏
11. Do you suffer from nausea or vomiting? ❏
12. Do you often have a bitter taste in your mouth or a furry tongue? ❏
13. Do you have a strong reaction to alcohol? ❏
14. Do you suffer from bloating? ❏
15. Does coffee leave you feeling jittery or unwell? ❏

Total Score

7 or more: If you answer yes to seven or more questions, you need to improve your detox potential.

4–6: If you answer yes to between four and six questions, you are beginning to show signs of poor detoxification and need to improve your detox potential.

Fewer than 4: If you answer yes to fewer than four questions, you are unlikely to have a problem with detoxification.

Anyone can benefit from the detox

If you have discovered that you are experiencing several of the symptoms listed above, you will benefit the most from my 9-Day Liver Detox, but the principles of the diet are also good for anybody who just wants to feel great. People who have followed the program often report that they now experience:

* Better energy
* A clearer mind
* Waking up alert and refreshed
* No more bloating
* A clear nose—not stuffed up

* No more bags or dark circles under the eyes
* Easier weight loss
* Better digestion
* Better and clearer skin
* No more water retention
* No more PMS
* Fewer aches and pains
* No more infections

To help you continue to enjoy better health, once you have completed the detox, which requires you to remove foods that can cause intolerances, I'll explain how to reintroduce those potentially offending foods and drinks to help you define your perfect diet for daily living.

How toxic are you?

Our bodies are permanently under assault from toxins. There are those outside our bodies that come from our environment, there are those that our own bodies make, and, of course, there are those toxins that we put into our bodies ourselves.

The liver is the clearing house for all these toxins. When it cannot process (detoxify) toxins fast enough because of overload, the toxins have to be stored in the body to be dealt with later. Guess where they are stored? In the fat cells. So we put on weight and inches not only because of our unhealthy eating habits but also to accommodate all these unprocessed toxins. When the liver is ready to cope with these additional toxins, they are released from the fat cells for processing and are transported via the lymphatic system (the transport system for fat molecules), the kidneys, and the blood. This makes it easier for your body to shed the weight and inches through healthy eating and exercise, because now the fat cells are not clinging to the toxins in an attempt to protect your body from their effects. When these toxins stay in the body, the whole system literally becomes *intoxicated*. Many hundreds of different symptoms and health problems can result from a liver that is having difficulty coping with excess toxins, including the ones illustrated in the diagram below.

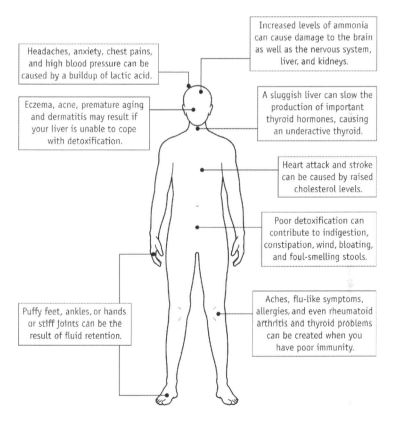

Problems that can result from a faulty liver

Skin complaints

Like the liver, the skin is also an organ of detoxification. When your liver isn't working optimally, your skin will try to eliminate toxins. This can cause a variety of unpleasant side effects, such as premature aging, acne, eczema, and dermatitis.

Poor digestion

Without bile, which is produced in the liver and stored in the gallbladder, you cannot digest fat. If fats are not being "emulsified"—that is, made water soluble—they will pass into the large intestine for elimination. Bile also stimulates peristalsis, which is the muscular movement of the digestive tract that propels food along it. A sluggish bowel results in constipation; when, finally, there is a bowel movement, the stool will contain greasy, undigested fat and will smell foul!

Fats are an important part of a healthy diet, and contained in them are the fat-soluble vitamins A, D, E, and K, which are essential for health. Signs of their deficiency include:

* Susceptibility to colds and infections
* Feeling run-down and tired
* Skin complaints
* Poor hair condition
* Bleeding gums
* Stress-related disorders
* Poor night vision
* A burning sensation in the mouth and throat
* Insomnia
* Lack of sex drive
* Exhaustion after light exercise

* Easy bruising
* Slow wound healing
* Varicose veins
* Poor skin elasticity
* Loss of muscle tone
* Infertility

Other unpleasant side effects of poor digestion include:

* Indigestion
* Bad breath
* Nausea
* Bloating
* Constipation and diarrhea
* Irritable bowel syndrome
* Weight gain

Poor immunity

The liver contains many immune cells that clean up debris from the blood as it travels through the liver for cleaning. When the liver is compromised and foreign particles flow back into the bloodstream, the immune system launches an attack. As a result, you are more likely to suffer from hard to shift infections, flu-like symptoms, allergies, and possibly even autoimmune diseases like rheumatoid arthritis and thyroid problems.

High cholesterol

The liver produces HDLs: high-density lipoproteins known as good cholesterol. They have an important job to do, traveling around the body collecting any excess cholesterol and transporting it out of the arteries and back to the liver. From there, it is taken away in bile and excreted in the stool. With poor bile flow, the cholesterol accumulates and your risk for a heart attack or stroke increases. It can also be reabsorbed in the gut unless you have consumed enough fiber.

Fluid retention

Almost all the proteins found in the blood are made in the liver. Among their many tasks, blood proteins, particularly albumin, help to maintain correct fluid balance. If you are experiencing fluid retention (such as unexplained weight gain; puffy feet, ankles, or hands; or stiff joints), it may mean that your liver is not processing proteins efficiently.

Ammonia poisoning

You may be familiar with the sharp, penetrating smell of ammonia. It's so strong that one waft of smelling salts under the nostrils can bring someone out of a faint. However, more than just a sniff of this toxic, reactive, and corrosive gas can cause serious illness or even be fatal.

All proteins are made up of amino acids, and when they are broken down, they release ammonia. This then travels to the liver for removal from the blood and conversion into urea, which is excreted in the urine. Ammonia is also released in the kidneys, but what isn't excreted in urine travels back to the liver. If the liver is overworked, ammonia conversion into urea slows down, leaving an "ammonia pool," which has to be released into the blood. You might think you would know if you had an ammonia overload. Of course, if it were that bad you would be very ill indeed, but just a slight excess in circulating ammonia can cause damage to the brain, nervous system, liver, and kidneys.

Lactic acid poisoning

Lactic acid is a toxin released from our cells when energy production is impaired because the liver has not been able to store enough B vitamins, due to overload. Excess lactic acid is very common in chronic fatigue syndrome and causes aching muscles after only a small amount of exertion. A buildup of lactic acid can also cause panic attacks, anxiety, headaches, brain fog, chest pains, and soaring blood pressure levels.

I hope that this brief tour of liver function has convinced you that this vital organ is worth looking after. You can start by giving it a holiday when you embark on my 9-Day Liver Detox.

The two sides of the detox coin

"What is food to one man is bitter poison to others," said Lucretius (99–55 BC), the Roman healer and philosopher, some two thousand years ago. But there are common substances that we all consume that promote our health and well-being, whereas there are others that we know adversely affect our health. We can call the good guys nutrients and the bad guys toxins—or antinutrients, if you prefer.

The two sides of detoxification are to decrease the toxins, which your body struggles to remove, and to increase the nutrients, which your body needs both to stay well and to improve your ability to detoxify the antinutrients.

What are toxins?

The single greatest toxin the body has to detoxify every second of every day is the product of oxidation, or oxidants. Oxidants can damage the cells in our bodies if they are allowed to remain, the same way that rust will damage iron if it is allowed to form.

Many of these oxidants originate within the body as a normal process of energy creation in the cells, as fats and glucose are "burned" with oxygen. That's how we stay alive, so oxidation is not intrinsically bad. It's the products of oxidation that can cause harm if not dealt with appropriately. But there are other oxidants that come to us from outside, either in our food or the air we breathe. For example, eating burned or fried food, breathing in exhaust fumes, or smoking cigarettes (including secondhand smoke) exposes us to oxidants. In fact, one single puff of a cigarette contains a trillion oxidants. These oxidants, regardless of source, are known as free radicals, and they are highly reactive chemicals that can cause a lot of damage to our cells if they are not neutralized properly. Fortunately, there are ways of neutralizing the free radicals (this is covered in chapter 3).

We all suffer from the effects of oxidants, but other toxins don't affect each of us in the same way. Finding out what is toxic for you is half the battle toward improved health and well-being. We can call whatever makes you feel worse an "intolerance." In some cases, it might be a substance that just overloads your detox potential, such as alcohol or caffeine (found in coffee and other caffeinated drinks). For some people, the tiniest amount of alcohol or caffeine makes them feel unwell, whereas others can tolerate large amounts. In any case, we all benefit from minimal exposure to substances that the liver has to detoxify, whether they come from external or internal sources, including:

* **Caffeine and alcohol** (see chapter 2).

* **High-meat diets** (and particularly burned meat, for example, barbecued meat; see chapter 2), which can alter the body's acid balance for the worse and cause inflammation.

* **Saturated and damaged fats,** which can damage cell membranes and are also a source of inflammation (damaged fats are discussed in chapter 2).

* **Salt,** which is a stomach irritant and is linked to gastric cancer, and which also raises blood pressure.

* **Processed foods** high in chemical additives and flavor enhancers, such as tartrazine and MSG, or preservatives such as benzoates.

* **Recreational and medicinal drugs,** which place an enormous load on the liver, especially painkillers.

* **Environmental pollutants,** which include cigarette smoke, exhaust fumes, paint fumes, pesticides and chemicals found in nonorganic foods, and heavy metals from dental materials and nonorganic foods.

It's best to avoid any of the above that you can and to minimize your exposure to the rest.

In other cases, your intolerance will manifest as an allergy, which means that your immune system attacks the substance in question, whether it's grass pollen, molds, yeast, wheat, or milk. Allergies come in different shapes and sizes, from full-blown immediate allergies (usually based on a kind of antibody called IgE attacking the offending item) causing instant reactions, to "hidden," or delayed, allergies (based on IgG antibodies). Many people have these without even knowing it, but feel worse as a result. My 9-Day Liver Detox eliminates the most common food allergens and shows you how to reintroduce foods to limit those that rob you of vitality. Of course, the best way to find out whether you have any allergies is to have a food intolerance test (see Resources).

How your liver detoxifies

If eating the right food is one side of the coin, detoxification is the other. From a chemical perspective, much of what goes on in the body involves substances being broken down, built up, and turned from one thing into another. A good 80 percent of this work in the body involves detoxifying potentially harmful substances. Much of this work is done by the liver, which represents a clearinghouse able to recognize millions of potentially harmful chemicals and transform them into something harmless or prepare them for elimination. This often means turning a fat-based toxin into something water soluble that can be eliminated in the urine. The liver is the chemical brain of the body, recycling, regenerating, and detoxifying in order to maintain your health.

The external toxins, or exotoxins, listed on pages 20 and 21 represent just a small part of what the liver has to deal with; many toxins are made within the body from otherwise harmless molecules. Every breath and every action can generate toxins. So, too, can and do the bacteria and yeasts that live inside us. These internally created toxins, or endotoxins, have to be disarmed and eliminated in just the same way that exotoxins do. If they are not eliminated, the body becomes irritated and inflamed. Antibodies formed to protect us against the harmful effect of potential toxins often trigger an autoimmune response, so our body actually starts fighting itself. If toxins can't be broken down, they are stored in the liver and in fat.

So, whether a substance is bad for you depends as much on your ability to detoxify it as on its inherent toxic properties. If your ability to detoxify is overloaded, you may have more toxins in your system, and on top of that, other key functions in the liver may be impaired: for example, the liver's ability to activate vitamins and minerals, which it needs to process if they are to be effective, or its ability to burn fat for energy. My 9-Day Liver Detox gives your liver a holiday as well as providing an eating plan and recommended supplements that help your liver detoxify any residual toxins. Let me explain why these foods and supplements help you detox.

Liver detoxification is a two-step dance

The ability of the liver to detoxify has two distinct phases. You can think of phase I as the preparation phase, where toxins are acted on by a series of enzymes (called P450). This phase converts toxins into a form that can be disarmed. Often, however, this process itself can produce unwanted by-products, or reactive intermediates, such as free radicals, that act as toxins. To avoid this phase I side effect there is a whole series of nutrients, particularly antioxidants, that you need to support your liver.

Detox nutrients: The phase I heroes

The first phase of liver detoxification (the gray area above the line in the illustration on page 24), which involves the P450 family of enzymes, mainly depends on having a great supply of antioxidant nutrients. These include:

Glutathione and/or **N-acetylcysteine,**[1] found in onions and garlic

Coenzyme Q10,[2] found in oily fish, spinach, and raw seeds and nuts

Vitamin C,[3] found in broccoli, peppers, citrus fruits, and berries

Vitamin E,[4] found in raw seeds, nuts, and fish

Selenium,[5] found in raw seeds, nuts, and fish

Beta-carotene,[6] found in carrots, peaches, watermelon, sweet potatoes, and butternut squash

These antioxidants are team players. You need all of them for your detox potential to be optimum. You may have seen newspaper headlines claiming that some recent research shows that antioxidants confer no benefits. This is because antioxidants are tested alone, whereas in fact they work best in synergy with

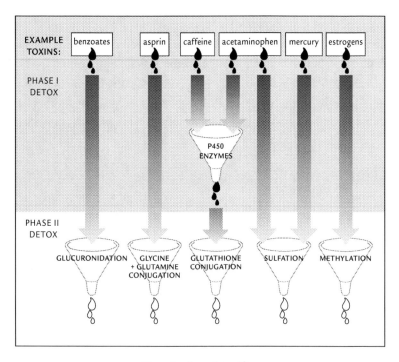

How the liver detoxifies

other antioxidants. For example, in one study beta-carotene given on its own to smokers had slightly increased their risk of cancer, but reduced the risk if given in combination with other antioxidants.[7] Vitamin E generally reduces your risk of heart disease as part of a multivitamin, but not if you take a large amount on its own with cholesterol-lowering statin drugs.[8] This is because cholesterol-lowering statin drugs knock out coenzyme Q10 (CoQ10), another natural anti-oxidant, which is vital for "reloading" vitamin E to detoxify another oxidant. Without enough CoQ10, vitamin E becomes an oxidant—a toxin in its own right. (See the diagram on page 68—"Antioxidants are team players"—to see how antioxidants work together.)

There are also various phytonutrients (substances from plants that have nutritional value) and herbs that can help. These include:

DIM (diindolylmethane), a substance in cruciferous veg-etables such as broccoli that helps detoxify excess estrogens and hormone-disrupting chemicals such as PCBs and dioxins as well as some herbicides and pesticides.[9]

Bioflavonoids,[10] including anthocyanidins in blueberries,[11] quercetin in red onions,[12] polyphenols in green tea,[13] and the herb milk thistle, which contains a powerful detoxifying nutrient called silymarin that protects liver cells from all kinds of toxins.[14]

Foods rich in these nutrients are included in my 9-Day Liver Detox Recipes, as well in the detox supplements I recommend (see page 110).

At phase II, the reactive intermediates are rendered non-toxic. This happens when enzymes link the toxin to another molecule that makes it more water soluble and less toxic. In this process, often called conjugation, the toxin is "married" to a key detoxifying nutrient. For example, the diagram below shows you how your body detoxifies acetaminophen, aspirin, and caffeine. (You'll see on page 79 how a simple urine test that involves taking a measured amount of caffeine, acetaminophen, and aspirin can determine your liver's detox capacity.)

The body processes toxins in the liver using different chemical pathways. Shown here are examples of what the liver does with caffeine, acetaminophen, or aspirin. These different pathways (for example, glutathione conjugation or sulphation) need different nutrients to work properly.

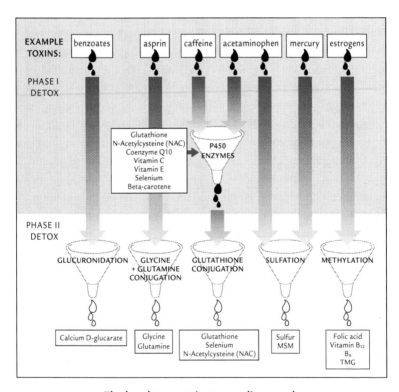

The key detox nutrients your liver needs

Detox nutrients: The phase II heroes

In phase II, the liver detoxifies substances by attaching things to them so that they are ready to be eliminated from the body in the process called conjugation, described above. There are five main ways in which the liver detoxifies.

Glucuoronidation. Possibly the most important detox pathway of all, it depends on calcium D-glucarate, which is found in apples, brussels sprouts, broccoli, cabbage, and bean sprouts.[15]

Glycine and glutamine conjugation. These are amino acids found in root vegetables and sprouts.

Glutathione conjugation. This pathway depends on a good supply of glutathione, an amino acid complex made from three amino acids (glycine, cysteine, and glutamic acid). Onions and garlic are a good source. Root vegetables are rich in glycine. The mineral selenium also helps glutathione work. Glutathione can be made in the body from N-acetylcysteine (NAC), a substance that is usually given in cases of acetaminophen overdose to trigger the liver into detoxifying.[16] Glutathione is recycled by anthocyanidins in berries as well as by alpha-lipoic acid,[17] so supplementing with both anthocyanidins (blueberries are particularly rich in these) and glutathione plus alpha-lipoic acid is much more powerful.

Sulfation. This depends on the sulfur-containing amino acids found in onions, garlic, and eggs. There's a type of sulfur you can supplement, called MSM, that helps the body detoxify.

Methylation. This key detoxifying process depends on B vitamins, especially folic acid (in greens and beans), vitamin B12 (animal source only), and vitamin B6, as well as trimethylglycine (TMG), once again found in root vegetables.

You don't need to know the chemistry, but you do need to know that each of these foods, rich in key detox nutrients, is included in the 9-Day Liver Detox Diet Recipes and daily menus. In addition, I also recommend taking specific detox nutrients to provide additional liver support (see page 72).

Maintaining the right balance

The final key factor in supporting the detoxification pathways is maintaining the right acid-alkaline balance in the body. The correct balance is one that is not too acid. When foods are metabolized by the body, a residue is left that can alter the body's acidity and alkalinity. Depending on the chemical composition of the metabolized foods ("ash"), the food is called acid-forming or alkaline-forming. However, this is not the same as the immediate acidity of a food. Oranges, for example, are acid due to their citric acid content, but citric acid is completely metabolized and the net effect of eating an orange is to alkalize the body, so oranges are classified as alkaline-forming.

Protein is made of amino acids, and is acid-forming. Foods such as fruits and vegetables are high in potassium and magnesium. These foods, as well as seeds and nuts, are also high in calcium. They have a more alkaline effect on the body, because the minerals they contain are alkaline. Your body can and does compensate, keeping the blood at the right pH; however, a diet excessively high in acid-forming foods is not good for you. Your 9-Day Liver Detox is more alkaline-forming, by virtue of including plenty of fresh fruit and vegetables in your diet. Roughly 80 percent of our diet should come from alkaline-forming foods, and 20 percent from acid-forming foods. The table on page 30 shows which foods are which.

Heal your digestive tract—
and take a load off your liver

Whereas your liver does most of the detoxing, effectively filtering and cleansing the blood of toxic material, your digestive tract, which represents a surface area the size of a tennis court, is the gateway between the food you eat and your bloodstream. It is actually the first line of detoxification, with the gut bacteria helping to neutralize unwanted microorganisms, while the digestive enzymes help to break down food into the right pieces to enter your body.

That tennis court inside you can be healthy or unhealthy. If it is unhealthy, it will become more permeable, which means that larger food particles not on the "guest list," so to speak, will get into the bloodstream, and this is called leaky gut syndrome. Whole food proteins, rather than their constituent amino acids, will gate-crash into your bloodstream, and your body's policemen—the antibodies—will attack, forming what is known as an immune complex. This is then treated by the body as a toxin and forms the basis of most food allergies and sensitivities, which have a detrimental effect on your overall health.

So, one immediate way to help detox your body is to improve the integrity of your digestive tract. You can actually test the "intestinal permeability" of your digestive tract (a nutritional therapist can advise you), but for now I'm going to recommend something much simpler: a teaspoon of glutamine powder.

The Glutamine factor—your gut's best friend

Although most of your body's organs are fueled by glucose, your digestive tract is a different story. It's a vast and highly active interface between your body and the outside world, and it needs a lot of fuel to work properly day in and day out. It

ACID, NEUTRAL, AND ALKALINE FOODS

High acid	Medium acid	Neutral	Medium alkaline	High alkaline
	Brazil nuts			Almonds
	Walnuts			Coconut
Edam		Butter		Milk
Eggs	Blue cheese			
Mayonnaise	Cheddar cheese		Avocados	Beans
		Coffee	Beets	Cabbage
Fish	Herring	Sugar	Carrots	Celery
Shellfish	Mackerel	Tea	Potatoes	Lentils
			Spinach	Lettuce
Bacon	Oats			Mushrooms
Beef	Rice			Onions
Chicken	Rye			Root vegetables
Lamb	Wheat			Tomatoes
Liver				
Veal	Cranberries		Dried fruit	Apricots
	Olives		Rhubarb	Apples
	Plums			Bananas
				Berries
				Cherries
				Figs
				Grapefruit
				Grapes
				Lemons
				Melons
				Oranges
				Peaches
				Pears
				Prunes
				Raspberries
				Tangerines

Acid ⟵――――――――――|――――――――⟶ Alkaline

runs on an amino acid called glutamine, thus sparing the glucose from your food for your brain, heart, and liver.

Not only does glutamine power your gut, it heals it as well. The endothelial cells that make up the inner lining of your digestive tract replace themselves every four days and are your most critical line of defense against developing food allergies or getting infections. As your "inner skin," your gut takes lots of hits: alcohol, nonsteroidal anti-inflammatory drugs (NSAIDs) such as aspirin and ibuprofen, antibiotics, coffee, and fried foods are some common gastrointestinal irritants. In Japan, people taking NSAIDs for pain and inflammation are also often instructed to take 2,000 mg of glutamine thirty minutes beforehand to prevent stomach bleeding and ulceration.

Many people suffer from digestive problems and possibly food allergies. My top tip (besides avoiding allergenic foods) is to take glutamine every day during your 9-Day Liver Detox, together with digestive enzymes and a probiotic supplement (see Resources). Glutamine is the preferred food of the cells lining the intestine, so I recommend one to two heaping teaspoons (that's 4,000 to 8,000 mg) of glutamine powder taken the last thing at night, diluted in a glass of water. This will help your gut to heal and rejuvenate.

Under normal circumstances, most of the glutamine in your food gets used up as fuel for your gastrointestinal tract. However, about 5 percent of it is used to make glutathione, the liver's most powerful antioxidant.

Glutathione, as we saw earlier, is made from three amino acids: glycine, cysteine, and glutamic acid, or glutamine. Think of them as the Three Musketeers. Glutamine is found in protein foods, such as beans, fish, chicken, and eggs, as well as in vegetables such as cabbage, spinach, beets, and tomatoes. Cysteine is a sulfur-containing amino acid found in onions, garlic, and eggs. And glycine is found plentifully in root vegetables. By getting more of each of these amino acids, you are providing yourself with the building blocks for glutathione, which boosts your liver and protects every single cell in your body from dangerous oxidizing chemicals, or free radicals.

So that's the end of your whistle-stop tour of how your body detoxifies. Now we will go on to discover the ways you can enhance your detoxification. The next two chapters give you the reasons and the ground rules behind the Six Golden Rules of your 9-Day Liver Detox: the five habits to break (explained in chapter 2) and the five habits to make (explained in chapter 3). These golden rules have all been taken into account in building our daily menus and recipes for you to follow.

Chapter Two

Five Habits to Break

To get the most powerful health transformation during your 9-Day Liver Detox, I am going to ask you to break five habits. These habits are the foods and drinks that most people enjoy to some extent but which will adversely effect your liver's detoxing process, as I will explain in this chapter. The five habits to break are:

1. Wheat
2. Milk
3. Caffeine
4. Alcohol
5. Bad fats

Wheat—our deadly bread

Bread may be a staple food for you, but for many it's more of a cereal killer than a staff of life. The reason is that wheat contains a protein called gluten, and specifically the component of gluten called gliadin, which is exceedingly unfriendly to your

digestive tract. As I explained in chapter 1, foods that the body
cannot digest can pass through the gut wall and are recognized
as toxins in the bloodstream, so it is important to avoid these to
allow the liver to focus on detoxifying the toxins that are already
present without introducing new ones. As your digestive system
is where detoxification starts, it's important to remove wheat
from your diet during your nine-day detox. However, as we
don't all react to wheat in the same way, it may not be necessary
for you to avoid wheat after the nine days is over.

Those people who are the most wheat-reactive will eventually have a digestive tract that is as flat as a pancake, because
all the tiny protrusions, called villi, which create the massive
surface area of your insides, will be literally destroyed. This is
called celiac disease and it affects approximately one in a hundred people (although many medical textbooks wrongly say
one in four thousand).[1] Far more people, and this may possibly
include you, have a lesser allergy or intolerance to wheat. So,
how do you know if you are one of them? There are two ways:
You can take a proper allergy blood test, or you can avoid wheat
for nine days and see how you feel. If you follow this second
course and find that you feel much better at the end of nine days,
but worse when you reintroduce it, I recommend you have a
blood test (see Resources for more details on allergy tests).

The common symptoms of gluten allergy
If you are suffering from any of these conditions, this may point
to a gluten allergy:

* Sniffling and snuffling, and sinus problems
* Fatigue and chronic fatigue syndrome
* Mouth ulcers
* Anemia

* Diarrhea or constipation
* Abdominal bloating
* Crohn's disease or diverticulitis
* Depression
* Poor concentration and brain fog

The problem protein: Gluten

Since you need to avoid allergens during your detox, some background about one of the most common ones may be helpful in understanding why wheat can be such a problem. Gluten is the key protein in wheat, but it's also found in rye, barley, and oats that have been processed on equipment also used for gluten-containing grains. In fact, gluten is a name for a family of proteins found in grains. The principal type of gluten, called gliadin,[2] is in wheat, along with glutenin, but rye and barley also contain chemically similar types of gluten (secalin and horedin respectively), so a person who is wheat sensitive is also likely to react to barley and rye. Oats are quite different, however, because the type of protein in oats bears no resemblance to gliadin. Approximately 80 percent of people diagnosed with celiac disease don't react to oats.[3]

About one in three people tested for IgG food allergy (see chapter 1) will react to wheat. Of these, 90 percent will react to gliadin, whereas 15 percent will react to barley and 2 percent will react to rye. Even fewer react to oats. Most people's immune systems react to gliadin when it gets into the bloodstream— and that may mean that you are affected. So this is why it's important to avoid wheat, as it may be recognized as a toxin in your system, as I will explain below. But first, at little about its history.

How it all began

When it comes to eating grains, this is a relatively new food for the human race. Humankind started eating gluten grains, at the earliest, ten thousand years ago. If the history of humankind were condensed into twenty-four hours, we would have been eating gluten grains for, at most, six minutes. Some cultures started eating wheat only in the last one hundred years—or the last two seconds. Thanks to advances in DNA research, we now know that we humans shrank in height when we shifted to a grain-eating peasant diet. Our hunter-gatherer ancestors, living on meat, fish and shellfish, vegetables, fruit, nuts, and seeds, were 5 to 6 inches taller, and had 11 percent larger brains.

All this history is encoded in your genes, and recently it has been discovered that gluten-allergic people have a genetic tag called DQ2 and DQ8, which has also been revealed to be increasingly common in societies that introduced grains late, including northwestern Europe, and especially western Ireland and Scandinavia, where grain growing isn't easy and consequently people's bodies have not adapted over the millennia to accept gluten grains.[4]

Why you might be sensitive to wheat

What this research is showing is that as many as one in three people in Britain may have a gluten sensitivity. Gluten is made of two proteins, gliadin and glutenin, found in wheat, and, to lesser extent, rye and barley. These are normally broken down into amino acids. Of course, if you don't eat wheat very often and have impeccable digestion and a super healthy digestive tract, that is what happens. But some of us who don't digest so well can end up with gluteomorphins in the blood,[5] which are wheat-based opioids that can make you crave wheat products.[6]

How it affects the detox

The reason for avoiding wheat (and preferably all gluten grains) is that if you are sensitive to it, the immune system will treat particles of wheat as a toxic invader and send antibodies to bind themselves to them, forming what is called an immune complex. Once that happens, the liver is tied up detoxifying the immune complex and is not dealing with your other toxins. Given that gliadin irritates just about anyone's gut if there is enough of it, I recommend that you strictly avoid all wheat, rye, and barley products, but not oats, for nine days to give your digestive system a break.

Gliadin grains to avoid

During your detox avoid breads, cakes, biscuits, cereals, pastas, or other foods made from any of these gluten grains:

Wheat

Spelt

Barley

Kamut (a cereal grain that is an ancient relative of modern durum wheat, but is higher in lipids, amino acids, vitamins, and minerals)

Triticale (a man-made hybrid of rye and wheat)

Nongliadin grains that you can enjoy

Instead, you can have bread, pasta, cereals, and other foods made from:

Oats

Amaranth (a South American gluten-free pseudograin, or false grain, because it comes from a broad-leaved plant and not a grass. It is high in protein, fiber, and some of the key dietary minerals.)

Buckwheat

Corn

Besam, or gram flour (ground dried chickpeas)

Millet

Quinoa

Rice

For example, you can have rice- or corn-based cereals, rice crackers, rice cakes, besam chapatis, buckwheat pancakes, rice or buckwheat noodles, and cornbread (as long as they contain no wheat flour), as well as rice or quinoa with your main meal. These may be new foods for you, so we're giving you loads of easy gliadin-free recipes to choose from.

Milk—it's a four-letter word

If I were still breast feeding at the age of thirty—from another species of animal—wouldn't you consider that rather strange? That is actually what we all do by drinking milk. Put that way, it may not be so surprising that our immune systems often react against milk, as if it were an alien substance not on the body's "guest list," and have difficulty digesting it. So, as we want to aid our digestion rather than add to its load during the detox, milk is out during your 9-Day Liver Detox.

What's wrong with cow's milk?

Cow's milk is the most common food allergy, any way you look at it. A classic IgE-based allergy to milk is the most common food allergy, and so too is hidden or delayed IgG food allergy to milk.

Logically, milk's status as a gut irritant and an allergen isn't surprising, since it is a highly specific food, containing all kinds of hormones designed for the first few months of a calf's life. Like wheat, it's also a relatively recent addition to the human diet. Our ancestors, after all, weren't milking buffalos. Once we have been weaned as children, approximately 75 percent of people (25 percent of people of Caucasian origin and 80 percent of Asian, Native American, or African origin) stop producing lactase, the enzyme that's needed to digest milk sugar, or lactose. Lactase deficiency, or lactose intolerance, leads to significant diarrhea, bloating, cramping, and excess gas—all of which can increase gut permeability and, as a result, place a greater detox load on the liver. Between eighteen months and four years after birth, most Asians, Hispanics, African-Americans, Native Americans, and Caucasians of southern European descent gradually lose lactase—one of many clues that the human body isn't designed to drink cow's milk, at least beyond early childhood.[7]

How will milk affect the detox?

It's not the lactose—the sugar in milk—that causes milk allergy, however. It's the protein. In other words, you can be either lactose intolerant, or milk-protein allergic, or both, and often lactose intolerance and milk allergy occur together. I recommend avoiding milk for the same reason as wheat: If you are sensitive to milk protein, the immune system will treat it as a toxic invader and antibodies will attach to it in something called an immune complex. Once that happens, the liver is tied up detoxifying the immune complex and is not dealing with your other toxins. As we have seen in chapter 1, in order for the detox to work effectively we must reduce the toxins we are eating or drinking wherever possible to allow the liver to concentrate on those toxins that are already present in our body. In addition, nonorganic milk can contain traces of the hormones and antibiotics normally fed to cattle, and the pesticide and fertilizer residues from their fodder, which also have to be detoxified in the liver.

Of course, most of us have been brainwashed since childhood by the milk marketeers into believing that milk is not only a necessary food but also almost a wonder food. With that knowledge, it might seem surprising that half the world, for example most of China and Africa, can survive, let alone thrive, without it. Milk is a reasonably good source of calcium, among other nutrients, but drinking milk certainly isn't the only way, or necessarily the best way, to achieve optimal nutrition. On top of that, the more you have, the greater your risk of a wide range of common diseases, including breast, prostate, and colorectal cancer.[8] You'll be getting plenty of calcium on your 9-Day Liver Detox from other foods, including seeds, nuts, and beans.

Signs of intolerance

The classic signs of milk allergy or lactose intolerance are:

* Asthma
* Bronchitis
* Chronic fatigue
* Depression
* Diarrhea
* Eczema
* Frequent infections
* Headaches or migraines
* Heartburn
* Hyperactivity
* Indigestion
* Poor sleep

* Rheumatoid arthritis

* Rhinitis and sinus problems

If you have some of these symptoms, notice what happens during your 9-Day Liver Detox. If your symptoms clear up, I recommend you investigate the possibility that you have a milk allergy. Milk is present in most cheeses, cream, yogurt, and butter, and is hidden in all kinds of food; sometimes it's called milk protein, whey (milk protein with the casein removed), or casein, which is the predominant type of protein—and the most allergenic—in dairy products. You'll be amazed at how many foods contain milk: from bread and cereals to packaged food and potato chips.

Milk products to avoid

Milk (including goat's or sheep's milk)

Cheese

Cream

Butter

Yogurt

Ice cream

Probiotic drinks

Anything with milk solids

Whey

Instead, we'll give you delicious recipes that happen to be dairy free.

Milk alternatives

You can enjoy the following alternatives to dairy:

Rice, almond, quinoa, or soy milk

Coconut milk, butter, or cream

Soy yogurt

Pumpkin-seed butter

Nonhydrogenated vegetable oil spreads

Cashew cream (made by blending cashews with rice milk)

Eggs

If you do feel much better after a period without dairy products, and worse when you reintroduce them, you'll find that there are many delicious alternatives, including soy ice creams and cheeses, and pumpkin-seed butter.

Caffeine—kick the habit

If the thought of giving up coffee causes a burst of hostility toward me, then the chances are you are currently addicted to caffeine. Of course, you will probably tell yourself that one cup of coffee can't harm you, that you've read all sorts of reports in the newspapers about coffee being high in antioxidants, and that you don't even believe you could stop for nine days—or want to. But I'm sorry to say that all of this is simply denial that you've become somewhat dependent on your caffeine fix and can't imagine functioning without it. Caffeine is also found in tea and in drinks such as Diet Coke and Red Bull.

How caffeine affects the detox

Now, I'm not asking you to quit caffeine forever. Just for nine days. The reasons are simple. First, the body treats caffeine as a toxin, and as we discussed earlier, we need to eliminate toxins from our diet while we follow the 9-Day Liver Detox to give our liver a chance to cleanse the system. Second, I have witnessed so many people experience a tremendous gain in energy, mental clarity, and improved mood just by stopping caffeine. Third, blood sugar balance is the long-term key to both energy and weight control, but you'll never achieve good blood sugar stability if you consume a lot of caffeine.

If you felt full of energy all the time, would you even want caffeinated drinks? If you do take caffeinated drinks to give you a pick-me-up, wouldn't you rather be naturally so full of energy that you don't need picking up? Think of this as a nine-day experiment.

How does caffeine work?

By understanding how caffeine works you'll understand why it's a no-no on your 9-Day Liver Detox. The main reason you probably drink caffeinated drinks is that the caffeine content boosts your mood and energy. It does this by blocking the receptors for a brain chemical called adenosine. The body makes adrenaline (the hormone that is secreted when we are under stress, in order to prepare our body for exertion: the "flight-or-fight response") from dopamine. We then normally break down dopamine and adrenaline to return to normal. Adenosine blocks dopamine breakdown, so the body ends up with more dopamine and, therefore, more adrenaline. So with all that adrenaline, no wonder you feel more alert, motivated, and stimulated! Although, of course, that extra adrenaline will make some people feel uncomfortable and jittery. The downside is that the body, unable to break down these stimulants, blocks its ears, so to speak, by shutting down receptors for dopamine and adrenaline, so you end up needing more adrenaline, and thus more caffeine. Caffeine reaches its peak concentration thirty to sixty minutes after consumption, after which it is inactivated by the liver, with only half its peak level left after four to six hours. However, during this time, the liver has to work very hard to detoxify the caffeine and is consequently not detoxifying your other toxins.

Caffeine is dehydrating

Have you noticed how you have to go to the bathroom more frequently after drinking tea or coffee? This is because caffeine is a diuretic; that is, it encourages the body to get rid of its fluids. But the one thing you don't want when detoxing is to get rid of fluids, because then the toxins will just be reabsorbed into the body. Instead, you need lots of water—but we will talk about that in chapter 3.

Caffeine is addictive

Research shows that consuming as little as 100 mg of caffeine a day can lead to withdrawal symptoms when you stop, including headache, fatigue, difficulty concentrating, and drowsiness.[9] It's worth knowing that while a small cup of instant coffee may contain less than 100 mg of caffeine, a large fancy coffee drink often contains as much as 500 mg—five times the "addictive" dose. Chemicals are used in manufacturing decaffeinated coffee, and in the end it still contains traces of caffeine, although usually less than 5 mg per regular cup, together with two other stimulants called theophylline and theobromine (which is the addictive substance in chocolate). It's better for you, but not perfect.

The classic withdrawal effects from caffeine are tiredness, low mood, headaches, anger, and irritability. Overnight withdrawal from caffeine can induce all these; however, headaches more commonly occur after a day off caffeine for regular consumers. Studies show that the energy levels of regular coffee consumers drop on withdrawal, but are usually higher after a week off coffee. However, when you follow your 9-Day Liver Detox, including taking the recommended supplements, you'll halve the time it takes to experience the energy gain and halve any symptoms of withdrawal.

Regular caffeine consumers are less alert on waking than nonconsumers; however, they become equally alert on consuming the equivalent of a cup of coffee.[10] So, basically, coffee is highly effective at removing the withdrawal effects of coffee! Hand steadiness is considerably worse for those who consume 250 mg a day—the equivalent of two fairly strong coffees.

Caffeine makes you more stressed and tired

At best, coffee has minor short-term mental and emotional benefits, but these are not sustained. A study published in the *American Journal of Psychiatry* observed fifteen hundred psychology students divided into four categories depending on their coffee intake: abstainers, low consumers (one cup or the equivalent a day), moderate (one to five cups a day), and high (five or more cups a day). On psychological testing, the moderate and high consumers had higher levels of anxiety and depression than the abstainers, and the high consumers had a higher incidence of stress-related medical problems, coupled with lower academic performance.[11]

In an Optimum Nutrition survey of fifty-five thousand people in the United Kingdom, the more caffeinated drinks a person consumed the more tired he or she was. The symptoms that most correlated with increasing caffeine consumption were loss of energy, reduced libido, joint stiffness, and, for women, menopausal symptoms.[12]

Coffee is also bad for your heart. Just one morning cup of coffee dramatically hardens your arteries, making blood vessels stiffer.[13] This is associated with an increased risk of heart attack and a good reason for older people, especially those with high blood pressure, to lower their intake. Coffee, more than tea, is also now well-known to increase homocysteine levels, one of the best predictors of heart attacks and strokes,[14] as well as a clear sign that your body treats coffee as a toxin. Drinking two cups of coffee a day significantly raises your homocysteine level, which compromises the ability of your body to detoxify itself. Decaffeinated coffee also raises homocysteine, about 50 percent as much as does caffeinated coffee, so this effect is not caused by caffeine alone. It's believed to be in part due to another chemical in coffee called chlorogenic acid, which is also found in high levels in decaf coffee.

Coffee also appears to cause inflammation in the body, as shown by the presence of key inflammatory markers in the blood. A study involving over three thousand people in Greece found that those consuming 7 fluid ounces of coffee—about two cups—had between 28 and 30 percent higher levels of each of three kinds of inflammatory marker compared to non–coffee consumers.[15] Inflammation is now recognized as the basis for many chronic degenerative diseases, such as cancer, arthritis, cardiovascular disease, and dementia, so it makes sense to reduce unnecessary exposure to inflammatory agents, particularly when they are also slowing down the liver. A simple measure of the liver's ability to clear caffeine from your system is a urine test that indicates how well your liver is detoxing (see page 79).

Caffeine disrupts normal sleeping

The other big problem area with caffeine is sleep. When you go to sleep, your melatonin levels increase. Melatonin is a hormone produced by the pineal gland in the brain when night falls, and one of its important functions is to make you feel sleepy. Melatonin levels start to rise two hours before sleep, then peak somewhere between 2 and 3 a.m. before starting to fall, preparing us to wake up. Research conducted at Tel Aviv University found that volunteers given regular coffee, compared to decaf, slept an average of two hours less and halved the amount of melatonin produced.[16] The melatonin-depressing effects of caffeine last up to ten hours, making it wise to avoid caffeinated drinks after midday.

Another vital job for melatonin is as an antioxidant in phase I detoxification (see pages 23 to 24 for other phase I detox nutrients). So, if you take in too much caffeine and suppress melatonin production, your liver can't detoxify so well. And finally, the body will naturally start to release stored toxins while you sleep, so if you are getting less sleep because of your caffeine intake, fewer stored toxins are being released from the fat cells to the liver. So you may lose out on some weight loss as well!

Have a break

These are all the reasons why you need to quit caffeine during your 9-Day Liver Detox. For die-hard addicts, the evidence of a harmful effect from drinking just one cup of coffee containing no more than 100 mg of caffeine is weak. But during these nine days, give yourself, and your liver, a break from caffeinated drinks, coffee, and black tea.

If you drink more than one cup of coffee or black tea a day, start cutting back before you begin the 9-Day Liver Detox; otherwise, you may have a lot of unpleasant withdrawal symptoms, such as headaches and nausea. These will pass after about twenty-four hours, but can make the detox a very unpleasant experience for that period. So give yourself the best chance and don't give up caffeine altogether until you are already down to only one cup a day.

Caffeine drinks to avoid

During your detox, avoid the following:

> Colas and diet colas
>
> Red Bull and other caffeinated drinks

All coffee, including decaf

Black tea

Instead, you can have up to two cups of weak green tea if you wish, using the same tea bag. Green tea is much higher in polyphenols and antioxidants and, by using the same tea bag, the caffeine you'll be consuming is minimized. Also high in antioxidants is rooibos (red bush) tea.

Alternative drinks

Instead of caffeinated drinks, enjoy the following:

Green tea (no more than two weak cups, as above)

Rooibos (red bush) tea

Red berry or rose hip teas

Lemon and ginger tea

Water

Juice (see page 150)

Alcohol—give it a break

During the liver detox we want to avoid any foods or drinks that will add to the toxins already in our system or that will give our liver extra work. Putting aside any benefits a glass of red wine may have for heart health, there is no question that alcohol taxes both your liver and gut. The more alcohol you consume, the more antioxidants you need. This is because alcohol is detoxified by the liver using a liver enzyme called alcohol dehydrogenase, but when you consume more alcohol than this enzyme can handle the liver will instead metabolize the alcohol to chloral hydrate, the same thing found in Mickey Finns or knockout drops. Normally, alcohol is metabolized to acetaldehyde by an enzyme called acetyldehyde oxidase, and, from there, to harmless chemicals that can be excreted from the body. But if this enzyme is overloaded or underfunctioning, you end up with too much circulating acetaldehyde. This very acidic and toxic substance leads to ketoacidosis—what we commonly refer to as a hangover: headache, nausea, mental and physical tiredness, and aching muscles. Acidosis occurs when the blood has become too acid, in this case through the toxic metabolites of alcohol. Acidosis is a cause of premature aging and osteoporosis and can lead to other disease states. It is a frequently reported finding in excess alcohol consumption.[17] The liver enzyme responsible for detoxifying alcohol depends on a good supply of antioxidant nutrients, especially vitamin C.

Yet, even before alcohol gets to the liver it has negative effects in the gut, where it acts as an intestinal irritant. This adds to the risk of increased intestinal permeability (see chapter 1, Heal your digestive tract), which in turn adds to the risk of allergic reactions to absorbed particles of incompletely digested food and to the ingredients in the alcoholic drink itself. For this reason, many beer and wine drinkers become allergic to yeast. About one in five people, on testing, have this sensitivity. In addition, wine drinkers may become sensitive to sulfites, which are added to grapes during the winemaking process to control their fermentation. Sulfites are also found in exhaust fumes, and the liver enzyme that detoxifies sulfites is dependent on molybdenum, a trace element that is frequently deficient in the diet. Organic, sulfite-free wines and champagne are better for you, and champagne has the added bonus of being yeast free.

Alcohol can also cause cancer

As well as increasing intestinal permeability, alcohol wreaks havoc on intestinal bacteria and has been reported to convert gut bacteria into secondary metabolites, which increase the proliferation of cells in the colon, initiating cancer. Alcohol can also be absorbed directly into the mucosal cells that line the digestive tract, and converted into aldehyde, which then interferes with DNA repair and promotes tumors. There is also evidence that alcohol increases the risk of mouth, pharyngeal, laryngeal, and esophageal cancers (in other words, affecting the body all the way down the gastrointestinal tract from the mouth to the intestines) and primary liver cancer. It probably also increases the risk of colorectal and breast cancer.[18]

Alcohol destroys nutrients

There is little question that alcohol acts as an antinutrient. While some forms of alcohol, such as stout or red wine, deliver a few nutrients, especially B vitamins, alcohol itself is a potent destroyer of these same nutrients. Chronic alcohol consumption leads to multiple deficiencies of nutrients, due to the alcohol destroying nutrients, as well as disturbing digestion and absorption, and it also suppresses the appetite. Along with the B vitamins, other nutrients are knocked out by alcohol, including vitamin C, magnesium, and zinc. Drinking alcohol with a meal also reduces the amount of zinc and iron the body can absorb from the food.

Once you start to become drunk from alcohol, you've exceeded your body's ability to detoxify. If, in addition, you already have increased gut permeability and perhaps an allergy to something in the drink, you're putting your body in for some punishment and may suffer cumulative ill effects on your health. You'll experience this as the dreaded hangover: nausea, headache, brain fog, or stomach upset. And, in due course, your capacity for alcohol and ability to avoid hangovers will diminish. If your hangover is bad enough, you'll probably take a painkiller or two. Both alcohol and painkillers tie up the liver's detoxification processes when they could be spring-cleaning your body. (We can work out how well your liver is functioning by giving you a measured amount of aspirin, acetaminophen, and caffeine, then collecting a urine sample; see page 79.)

Alcohol is dehydrating

In just the same way as caffeine, alcohol is a diuretic, encouraging your body to get rid of its fluids. Without sufficient fluids, your toxins will be reabsorbed into the body. So, it's important to have no diuretics while detoxing.

The above reasons are why there's no alcohol during your 9-Day Liver Detox. Once it's over, I hope you will have a better functioning liver and digestive system and that you will continue to follow my "optimum nutrition" principles. So, a glass of wine or beer once or up to three times a week is unlikely to have a negative impact on your health. (But choose organic when you can.) If, on the odd occasion, you drink more, take vitamin C and other antioxidants beforehand, drink plenty of water along with the alcohol, have a teaspoon of glutamine powder (see page 29) in water before you go to sleep, and exercise the next day. All this will help to minimize the damage.

Alternative drinks

Instead of alcoholic drinks, enjoy the following:

Diluted fruit juice

Mineral water

Tomato juice

Fruit smoothies

Bad fats—stay away from bad trans and hydrogenated fats

There was a time when fats were just thought of as fuel for the body. But now we know that there are good fats and bad fats. The good fats are called omega-3 and omega-6 fatty acids, and we need to get them from our diet. The richest sources of essential fats are raw nuts, seeds and their oils, and oily, or carnivorous, fish such as salmon, mackerel, herring, and tuna. Sardines are good, too.

The bad fats are damaged fats. These are called trans fats, which these days are much in the news; some British supermarkets are even working to banish them from their own brand products. These damaged fats are found in deep-fried foods and some foods containing hydrogenated vegetable oils. So, if you want to minimize your exposure to trans fats, limit your intake of fried, and especially deep-fried, foods, and don't buy foods containing hydrogenated fats. Check the list of ingredients in processed foods: if a food has the "H" word in the ingredients, don't put it in your basket!

Why are trans fats so bad for you?

After you eat trans fats, they can be taken directly into the brain, where they disturb thinking processes by blocking the conversion of essential fats into vital brain fats such as GLA (gamma-linolenic acid), DHA (docosahexaenoic acid), and prostaglandins. Twice as many trans fats appear in the brains of people deficient in omega-3. So, a combined deficiency in omega-3 fats and an excess of trans fats is bad news indeed. In a typical junk food diet, up to a quarter of fat intake can be these damaged trans fats, which are found in a diet high in French fries, deep-fried foods, doughnuts, and other fast and convenience foods. Trans and hydrogenated fats are difficult to digest and slow to detoxify, clogging up the liver for long periods when it could be dealing with your other toxins.

On top of this, eating fried foods, especially deep-fried foods, or any "crisp" fat—such as bacon or browned cheese—delivers a large quantity of oxidants that your body has to detoxify with antioxidants. Your 9-Day Liver Detox avoids all these foods.

Is meat suitable for the diet?

Meat isn't necessarily bad news, however, as long as it's lean, organic, and unburned. But most meats, especially processed meats, are high in fats, and if the meat is burned, these become damaged fats. Many people think that white meat is better for you largely because it's lower in fat. But this really does depend on the animal and how it has been reared and fed. The average chicken in the 1970s had 9 grams of fat. Today, however, the average chicken is virtually obese, with 22 grams of fat. So, in this case, lean pork would be lower in fat than a fat chicken. That having been said, my recommendation for these nine days is to avoid all meat except seafood—be it red or white. We provide delicious meat–free recipes, so this is easy to do.

Fats to avoid

During your detox, avoid the following:

All meat (except seafood)

Fried fish and eggs

Processed foods with hydrogenated fats

Processed fat spreads

French fries and other fried vegetables

However, you do not have to avoid all fats, because those from nuts, seeds, and fish contain the essential omega-3 and omega-6 fats that are vital for your health. Seeds and nuts from plants that are grown in a hot climate (sesame and sunflower, for example) are rich sources of omega-6 fats, whereas seeds from a cold climate (walnut and flax, for example) are high in omega-3 fats. But there's a particularly potent couple of omega-3 fats, called EPA (eicosapentaenoic acid) and DHA, that are especially rich in coldwater fish with teeth—in other words, fish that eat fish: salmon, mackerel, herring, and tuna. It's vital to have the right amount and balance of these fats, which is why they are built into your 9-Day Liver Detox. In addition, I also recommend that you take a daily omega-3 supplement containing EPA and DHA (see page 72).

Alternative foods you can enjoy

Try these health-giving foods during your detox (and beyond):

Baked, poached, or steamed oily fish

Poached, boiled, or lightly scrambled eggs

Homemade mayonnaise

Raw nut and seed spreads, such as tahini or pumpkin-seed butter

Raw nuts and seeds

Raw cold-pressed nut and seed oils—for cold use only, such as in salad dressings or drizzled on vegetables after cooking

Also, you can use steam-frying instead of frying to give foods a good flavor (see page 109).

Chapter Three

Five Habits to Make

To be sure of maximum health at all times, it's well worth forming some good habits. I'm going to ask you to adopt some during your 9-Day Liver Detox and urge you to continue with them after your detox has finished, as they will maximize your energy and well-being. The five habits to make are:

1. Drink eight glasses of water each day
2. Eat the big five superfoods every day
3. Maximize your intake of antiaging antioxidants
4. Take detoxifying supplements
5. Do detoxifying exercises every day

Drink eight glasses of water each day

Drinking eight glasses of water—about 48 fluid ounces, or eight 6-ounce glasses—makes an enormous difference to how you feel, especially in your energy and mental clarity. Water helps to dilute toxins in the blood for elimination via the kidneys, so drinking water helps your kidneys to function better. Your water intake can include caffeine-free teas and coffee alternatives. (Caffeine is a diuretic, so it causes more water loss from the body.) So, this might mean having three hot drinks, your special "detox juice," and four glasses of water a day. Half a lemon squeezed into a mug of hot water is another good option, as lemon is a great antioxidant detoxifier and helps the liver flush its toxins into the bowel. You can also add a slice of ginger (another excellent antioxidant) as well as, or instead of the lemon, if you prefer.

However, 48 fluid ounces of water a day is really a minimum, because if the weather is hot, or if you exercise, you will need more water to replace the liquid you are losing as sweat.[1] Also, drinking more is generally helpful for the kidneys, because many toxins, both those generated by the body and those consumed, are eliminated via the kidneys. Drinking plenty of water helps dilute the concentration of toxins in the blood, so the kidneys have an easier time—up to a point. It's also important to keep your body hydrated so that toxins are not reabsorbed into your body from the bowel. The maximum amount of liquids drunk should be equal to the amount the kidneys can reasonably excrete in twenty-four hours, and in adults this is about 4 1/4 pints per day.[2] So, be aware that drinking more than you need, which is about 3 1/4 to 4 1/4 pints a day under normal circumstances, isn't better for you and may be worse. This is because too much liquid does tax the kidneys and can lead to overhydration. Taken to the extreme this can kill you—a man died after drinking 21 pints in an hour.

What happens if you don't get enough?

Water has many roles throughout the body other than flushing the kidneys, including dissolving minerals and acting as a delivery system, a lubricant, and a temperature regulator. Even very mild dehydration can lead to constipation, headaches, lethargy, and mental confusion, while increasing the risk of urinary tract infections and kidney stones.[3] When just 1 percent of body fluids are lost, body temperature goes up and mental concentration becomes more difficult.

The thirst mechanism kicks in when we have lost between 1 and 2 percent of body water. However, the thirst reflex is often confused with hunger. If we ignore it or mistake it for hunger, dehydration can continue to about 3 percent, where it seriously affects both mental and physical performance. Sports nutritionists have found that a 3 percent loss of body water results in an 8 percent loss in muscle strength. So, here are some tips to get you in the habit of drinking enough water:

* Drink a glass of water **when you wake up**. The blood and urine have the highest concentration of toxins in the morning, so drinking water helps you detoxify by diluting these toxins.

* Always drink **before you eat**. We often mistake thirst for hunger. So, especially if you are looking to lose weight, drink a glass of water before you reach for a snack or have a main meal.

* Drink two glasses of water **after you exercise**. Muscles get stiff when you exercise, and you also lose water through sweat. You need about 1 1/4 pints of fluids an hour, depending on the intensity of the exercise.

* **Keep water where you are.** Buy yourself an attractive 1-quart jug to keep on your desk at work. Fill it up with filtered water in the morning and drink it by the evening. Or buy 1 quart of natural mineral water and drink it by the evening. Alternatively, travel with a water container; fill it up, and drink it all, each day. One quart of water equals a little more than five 6-ounce glasses.

* Drink filtered or natural mineral water. Avoid any bottled water that isn't labeled "natural mineral water," even if it says "spring" or "pure." Only springwater that comes from a pure source and has consistent mineral levels season by season, year after year, can be labeled "natural mineral water." What this means is that the water fell to earth, often hundreds of years ago, and was then gradually pushed to the surface by underwater springs through deep bedrock cracks, purified and mineralized in the process. This water doesn't have any of the pesticide or nitrate contaminants found in the water table, and therefore in tap water.

Good water

The best water filters use carbon filtration systems fitted under the sink to give you purified water. I prefer these to distilled water or reverse osmosis, which remove all of the minerals in the water.

By the way, there's nothing wrong with naturally carbonated water. Carbon grabs ahold of minerals. Naturally carbonated mineral water such as Perrier, therefore, contains carbonated minerals that are absorbed into the body. However, the carbon in artificially fizzy drinks can grab hold of minerals in the body and take them out. People who drink lots of fizzy drinks, especially if they also contain phosphoric acid, tend to have less bone density as a result. So, the best mineral water to drink is naturally carbonated, followed by still, followed by artificially carbonated. Pure distilled water, while good from the point of view of containing no impurities, also contains no minerals. Most natural water contains significant amounts of minerals—for example 60 to 100 mg of calcium in 2 quarts of water. So, if you drink only distilled water, make sure you are getting all the minerals you need from your diet and supplements. Most important of all, whatever kind of water you drink, make sure you drink enough.

Signs that you don't drink enough

Any combination of the symptoms below might help you become more in tune with your body's cries for water:[4]

* Are you prone to constipation?
* Are you often thirsty?
* Do you have joint problems?
* Do you feel tired?
* Are you having difficulty concentrating?
* Are you overheating?
* Do you have dry skin, mouth, or lips?
* Do you get frequent infections?
* Do you have dry, brittle hair?

The other way to judge is the color of your urine. If your urine is very strongly colored, then you're not drinking enough water. This simple gauge is, however, complicated by the fact that riboflavin (vitamin B2) makes the urine a fluorescent kind of yellow. (Riboflavin is found in mushrooms, cabbage, broccoli, and mackerel, and is more likely to affect the urine color if you are also taking B vitamin supplements. This color in urine shows that you are taking in adequate amounts of riboflavin.) However, it is different from the dark yellow of urine that is too concentrated due to lack of water and is easy to recognize once you get used to it. Ideally, your urine should be a light, straw-colored yellow. If, however, your urine is often clear, like water, you may be drinking too much and would therefore not be taking in enough nutrients.

Eat the big five superfoods every day

Superfoods are simply foods that press all the right health buttons: they are packed with nutrients and antioxidants, and free from anything bad for you, including too much natural sugar. Since the goal of your 9-Day Liver Detox is to make sure everything you eat is packed with nutrients that support your liver's ability to detoxify, and is totally free from toxins, one of the simplest ways to take a step toward this goal is to set yourself the rule of five superfood portions a day. Now, we've built this into your nine-day menu, so you don't need to do anything, but if you want to improvise or just want to know why they are included in my 9-Day Liver Detox, read on.

1. Seeds of life

Everything grows from a seed. For this simple reason seeds are jam-packed full of energy, protein, and the nutrients necessary for plants to grow, and we grow from eating plants. All seeds are packed with minerals, such as calcium, magnesium, manganese, molybdenum, zinc, and selenium, all of which are essential for detoxification, but some seeds have more of one mineral than others. Pumpkin seeds are the highest in magnesium. Hot-climate seeds, such as sesame and sunflower, are high in the essential omega-6 fats that help to balance hormones and keep your skin healthy, whereas cold-climate seeds, such as flax, are higher in omega-3, vital for the health of your arteries, joints, and brain.

These seed nutrients (especially vitamin E, magnesium, manganese, molybdenum, and zinc) are especially important for the phase I detoxification described on page 24. In fact, zinc is essential for the phase I detoxification of alcohol, so you might consider supplementing before a night out! All these minerals, with the addition of selenium, are essential for manufacturing many of the conjugation enzymes in phase II detoxification. In addition, the essential fats in seeds speed up the time it takes for stools to be moved along the gut before a bowel movement, so that fewer toxins are absorbed or reabsorbed from the gut into the bloodstream.

Using a combination of these seeds provides the best all-around superfood (but please don't buy roasted seeds, or you will lose much of their benefit). You need a mixture of half flaxseeds, and half sesame, sunflower, and pumpkin seeds. This is what I call my Essential Seed Mix (see page 116 for how to prepare this). This gives the correct balance of minerals and omega-3 and omega-6 essential fats, and it tastes great. Mix these seeds together and keep in an airtight container in the fridge. No light, no heat, and no extra exposure to oxygen will keep them fresher for longer. Grind them as you need them in your now-unused coffee grinder—this allows you to get the most nutrients out of the seeds. In case you are wondering, they won't make you fat. Your 9-Day Liver Detox will contain a tablespoon of this Essential Seed Mix per day.

Essential Seed Mix

Have a tablespoon every day of ground seeds. Seeds are incredibly rich in essential fats, minerals, vitamin E, protein, and fiber

---

2. Go for greens

There's something special about dark green vegetables. They are packed with vitamin C, folate, and chlorophyll, all of which are exceedingly good for you. To give you an example of the benefits of folate, Dr. Jane Durga from Wageningen University in the Netherlands asked 818 people aged from fifty to seventy-five to take part in some research. Over a period of three years, she gave some of the group a supplement containing 800 mcg of the B vitamin folic acid a day (called folate in food)—which is what you'll receive every day on your 9-Day Liver Detox—and gave the others a dummy pill. On memory tests, the supplement users had scores comparable to people $5^1/_2$ years younger![5] As well as the benefits of folate, eating vitamin C–rich foods is linked to better skin, better energy, and a substantially lower risk of cancer.[6]

Of course, these are only three of dozens of vital nutrients found in greens, but some greens are better than others. Spinach is the highest in folic acid, giving 204 mcg in a cup, or a good handful, which is what you'll be having every day. Other great sources are watercress, basil, and parsley. You'll be having a handful of each of these in my Super Greens Mix, giving you 800 mcg a day—enough to give your memory a definite boost.

Also excellent is avocado, which you can add to the Super Greens Mix for a thicker consistency. During the detox, you'll be adding the Super Greens Mix, blended, to soups, salads, and other savory foods. We'll show you how on page 129. All you need is a blender.

Watercress, parsley, and basil are exceptional sources of beta-carotene (second only to carrots) and great sources of vitamin C (second only to broccoli and green peppers). All these super greens are packed full of bioflavonoids, which are special antioxidants that help your liver to detox your body. The combination is quite delicious and can be adapted to make pesto, soups, stews, and salads.

Super Greens Mix

Have a serving every day of our Super Greens Mix (see page 129 for how to prepare this): a blend of a handful each of baby spinach leaves, watercress, parsley, and basil with variations, such as sun-dried tomatoes, artichoke hearts, pine nuts, pumpkin seeds, and avocado.

3. Cruciferous vegetables rule

Vegetables whose leaves grow as a cross (cruciferous) are all part of a special food family that enhances the liver's capacity to detoxify. This includes cabbage, cauliflower, broccoli, brussels sprouts, and kale. They are good for us because they contain glucosinolates and D-glucarate, which help a critical liver detox process called glucuronidation. To illustrate this, some ingenious scientists managed to extract the glucosinolates from brussels sprouts and fed volunteers either regular brussels sprouts that still contained glucosinolates, or those with it extracted. Those fed the glucosinolate-containing brussels sprouts had a 30 percent more active antioxidant-enzyme function, showing just how powerful these glucosinolates are.[7] That's why I recommend them, and, if you follow the recipes and menu plans, you'll be having a serving of cruciferous vegetables every day.

Cruciferous Vegetables

Have a serving of broccoli, brussels sprouts, cabbage, cauliflower, or kale every day.

4. Sulfur so good

Onions, green onions, garlic, and shallots are excellent food sources of sulfur-containing amino acids. Sulfur drives a critical liver detox pathway called sulfation. The amino acids in these foods also give the body the raw ingredients to make glutathione, which drives another critical detox pathway. (You may recall that acetaminophen and caffeine are detoxified by glutathione, page 24.) Red onions are especially good because they are high in quercetin, which is a natural anti-inflammatory, curbing allergic reactions and pain.

Garlic has many other benefits, a key one being as a gut protector. It's a natural antifungal agent, thereby helping to keep your digestive tract free of unwanted fungi and yeast.

Sulfur-Up Your Diet

Have a garlic clove, a small onion, a shallot, or four green onions every day.

---

5. Get juicy

I want you to have a superjuice every day made from superfruits. Superfruits are high in antioxidants to support your liver, high in folic acid (which helps methylation, one of the most vital detoxification processes), high in zinc (vital for health and detoxification), and low in sugar. Blueberries, strawberries, and raspberries are the best all-around foods for antiaging antioxidants compared to other fruit. A serving of strawberries contains more antioxidant power than three apples or four bananas. Best of all are blueberries, which are especially rich in a type of flavonoid called anthocyanidins and proanthocyanidins. You can measure the total antioxidant power of a food by its ability to detoxify oxygen radicals (oxidants). This is called the ORAC (oxygen radical absorption capacity) score. The higher the score, the more potent the antioxidant. Berries come out on top, but there are other good fruits, too, including oranges, grapes, and watermelon.

Fruits	Zinc	Folic acid	ORAC	Vitamin C	Total ORAC score
Strawberries	4	3	4	5	21
Raspberries	2	3	4	5	19
Blueberries	3	5	5	1	19
Watermelon	5	2	3	4	18
Grapefruit	0	4	3	5	16
Oranges	0	4	3	5	15
Grapes	4	5	2	2	14

The top antioxidant fruits

We've devised a selection of superfruit smoothies based on these fruits for you. For example, there's the Berry Tasty (page 158), made with a handful of berries plus tahini, or my favorite, Watermelon Whiz (page 158), made simply by blending the flesh and seeds of a watermelon. The seeds crack and the black husks of the seeds sink to the bottom; the seed itself, which is rich in zinc, selenium, vitamin E, and essential fats, becomes part of the drink with the vitamin C– and beta-carotene-rich flesh. When berries are out of season, you can use frozen berries; otherwise it's best to pick fresh, organic fruits.

Add some carrot!

Although not a fruit, carrots are good combined with fruits for juices and smoothies. Carrots are great for you, and delicious with some apple or pear, and with ginger. Ginger is good for the digestion and a natural anti-inflammatory food. Try our Stomach Settler (page 156), made with carrot, pear, ginger, lemon juice, and a little pineapple, which contains the digestive enzyme bromelain.

You can also make vegetable juices if you prefer, but ideally have a juice containing carrot and a juice containing berries or watermelon on alternate days if you haven't eaten these foods already during the day (we have added a reminder on your menu plan for each day).

Why make juices and smoothies?

The advantage of juicing or blending over actually eating the fruit or vegetable is that you can consume a greater variety—and variety is really the key to antioxidants. They work best when you take many different ones together. If you didn't juice, you would have to eat an awful lot of different fruits and vegetables to get the same level of plant nutrients. There are other advantages too: Would you ever consider eating raw broccoli? Probably not, but it is a powerhouse of nutrients to support phase II detoxification, and it is far more concentrated in its raw state than if it were cooked. A few stems of raw broccoli (or, preferably, broccolini) can be juiced easily or blended, and it combines well with carrot and celery to make a delicious drink. Furthermore, if you use a blender, you can include parts of the fruit or vegetable that would otherwise be thrown away, such as the seeds and rind, where these amazing nutrients are most concentrated. If the end result is too thick to be a proper juice, then have it as a cold soup with a drizzle of organic yogurt and a sprig of mint. Think gazpacho.

> ### Drink a Superfood Juice or Smoothie Every Day
> Choose from our menu of delicious smoothies, including berries, watermelon, and citrus fruits (see pages 150 to 159).

Sugar in fruit

You might have noticed that the government guidelines on eating five portions of fruit and vegetables a day say that fruit juice counts as only one portion. This is because of the high sugar content of many fruits, particularly bananas, bearing in mind that the typical American diet is already very high in sugar. However, your detox lasts only nine days, and you will have removed your other sources of sugar during this time. Also, I believe the benefits of the vitamins and minerals contained in the fruit outweigh the temporary downside of the fruit sugar. But if you prefer not to add to your sugar load, avoid banana and stick to berries, or make it a vegetable juice.

Maximize your intake of antiaging antioxidants

I talked in chapter 1 about the potential damage caused by oxidants (free radicals), and I also mentioned that we have the means of neutralizing them. This is where antioxidants come in. Some of these are made in the body, and others are provided in our food. You've probably heard of the main food-derived antioxidants already: vitamin A (beta-carotene), vitamin C, vitamin E, zinc, and selenium—and there are many others. Many of the steps you'll take on your 9-Day Liver Detox will greatly increase your intake of antioxidants, and the recipes and menus we have created take your antioxidant intake from food to the max.

Antioxidants are team players, as you can see in the illustration below, which shows how your body would disarm the oxidant from a French fry. It would need vitamin E (from seeds and fish), coenzyme Q10 (mainly made in the body), vitamin C (from fruits and vegetables), glutathione (from onions and garlic), and anthocyanidins (from berries), with some beta-carotene (from carrots or watercress) and some alpha-lipoic acid (made in the body) thrown in. Now you understand why these foods are all part of your 9-Day Liver Detox.

How the antioxidants work

To explain how antioxidants work, we can compare an oxidant to a hot potato. The antioxidant then, vitamin E, for example, is like an oven glove that stops the oxidant from burning you. However, the antioxidant becomes hot in the process and itself becomes an oxidant. Ultimately, if you've got enough nutrients

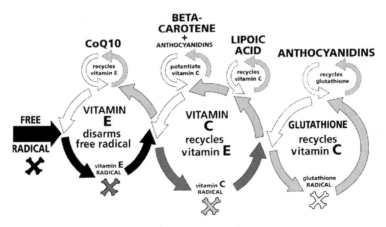

Antioxidants are team players
A fat-based oxidant, technically called a free radical, can be disarmed by vitamin E. The vitamin E molecule then becomes an oxidant, or free radical, and is in turn disarmed and put back to work by vitamin C and CoQ10.

you'll quench the oxidant and reload the antioxidants to go back to work ready to disarm the next oxidant.

The box on page 70 lists the top twenty antioxidant-rich foods, as rated on the ORAC (oxygen radical absorption capacity) scale. Make sure you eat five of the twenty foods each day.

Take detoxifying supplements

In chapter 1, you learned about a whole host of nutrients that make phase I and phase II of liver detoxification work best. While the 9-Day Liver Detox will work in its own right, you can further improve and support your liver's ability to detoxify by supplementing the right combination of nutrients. On page 72, I recommend supplements for you to take only during your detox. You don't need to take them every day once the detox is over.

My first recommendation is to supplement a combination of digestive enzymes, probiotics, and glutamine. Digestive enzymes help digest your food, minimizing the chances of whole food proteins getting into the blood. Probiotics are essential beneficial bacteria, which also play a part in the digestive process. I like the strains *Lactobacillus acidophilus* and *Bifidobacteria*. You don't need these every day of your life, but a nine-day course is a great way to repopulate your gut flora, or "inner garden." The combination of digestive enzymes plus probiotics, available in some supplements, is like a day at a health spa for your insides (see Resources).

My second recommendation is a teaspoon of glutamine powder last thing at night to help maintain the integrity of the gut wall, your first line of defense from toxins (see Resources). Glutamine is direct fuel for the gut lining.

The top 20 Antioxidant Power Foods

All foods are in ORAC units per 100 grams (the higher the
units the higher the antioxidants).

1.	Pomegranate	3,037
2.	Blueberries	2,234
3.	Blackberries	2,036
4.	Kale	1,770
5.	Strawberries	1,536
6.	Raspberries	1,227
7.	Baby spinach, raw	1,210
8.	Broccoli (or, preferably, broccolini)	1,183
9.	Plums	949
10.	Alfalfa sprouts	931
11.	Spinach, steamed	888
12.	Beets	841
13.	Avocado	782
14.	Orange	750
15.	Grapes, red	739
16.	Peppers, red bell	731
17.	Cherries	670
18.	Kiwifruit	602
19.	Beans, baked	503
20.	Grapefruit, pink	483

My third recommendation is an all-around antioxidant or
liver-support formula (see Resources). Pick the formula that has
the greatest number of the key liver-support nutrients shown
below:

* Vitamin C

* Vitamin E

* Coenzyme Q10

* Glutathione
* N-acetylcysteine
* Alpha-lipoic acid
* Glycine
* Glutamine
* Calcium D-glucarate
* Milk thistle (silymarin)
* DIM (diindolylmethane, broccoli extract)
* MSM (a form of sulfur)
* Trimethylglycine (TMG)

In addition, you need B vitamins that help methylation, but you'll find these, as well as basic levels of antioxidants plus minerals, in a high-potency multivitamin-multimineral. I recommend everyone to take three basic supplements every day:

* A high potency multivitamin-multimineral (good ones have 5 mg zinc and 100 mg magnesium)
* One gram of vitamin C, plus bioflavonoids found in berry extracts
* Essential omega-3 (EPA and DHA) and omega-6 (GLA) fats

Very rarely I have come across someone who is in such toxic overload that supplements and herbs can cause a bad reaction, such as headaches or nausea. If this is the case for you, then stop taking any supplements and just focus on the other food recommendations. You may have to do my 9-Day Liver Detox a couple of times before your body can tolerate the supplements.

Take detox supplements every day

Your daily supplement program should look like this:

	DOSAGE		
	Breakfast	Lunch	Dinner
During the 9-Day Liver Detox			
Digestive enzymes/ probiotics/glutamine	1	1	1
Glutamine powder			1 tsp at bedtime
Antioxidant/liver-support formula	1	1	
Every day			
High-potency multivitamin	1	1	
Vitamin C	1	1	
Essential fats (EPA, DHA, and GLA)	1		

Do detoxifying exercises every day

Detoxification is about eliminating what is unnecessary. This is not only a process that happens in your body but also a process for your mind and the environment you live in. In chapter 1, I talked about unprocessed toxins being stored in the fat cells and eventually being released, detoxified, and removed from the body via the blood, kidneys, gut, and also the lymphatic system. The lymphatic system carries fats absorbed from food into the circulation and carries cellular waste (including stored toxins) to the liver for detoxification, so its efficient functioning is vital for your 9-Day Liver Detox. Unlike the cardiovascular system, which includes the heart, the lymphatic system doesn't have a pump and relies on movement to help detoxify. That's why breathing and physical exercise that stimulate lymphatic drainage help detoxification.

But exercise has another important role to play, and that is the generation of vital energy, called qi in Chinese medicine and ki in Japan. Any whole-body exercise is good for detoxification (brisk walking, jogging, swimming, yoga, and so on) but my favorite vital-energy-generating exercise is Psychocalisthenics, because it combines both movement and qi-generating breathing.

Psychocalisthenics is a precise sequence of twenty-three exercises that leaves you feeling fantastic. I've been using it for twenty years, and I've yet to find anything that makes me feel better—which isn't bad for fifteen minutes a day! Each exercise is driven by the breath, leaving you feeling lighter, freer, and thoroughly oxygenated after a simple routine that anyone can do. At first glance, it looks like a powerful kind of aerobic yoga. Psychocalisthenics is designed to generate both physical fitness and vital energy by bringing mind and body into balance. Its key lies in the precise breathing pattern that accompanies each physical exercise.

The best way to learn Psychocalisthenics is to do a short course. You can also teach yourself from a DVD, but it is best to learn it in a class (see Resources).

Alternatively, join a yoga class that teaches breathing techniques and combine this with physical exercise such as walking for twenty minutes a day for a similar effect.

Detoxifying breathing and meditation
Another way to generate vital energy is with meditation. This also helps to clear and detoxify the mind of endless thoughts. If you are new to meditation, I recommend a very simple breathing exercise, called Diakath Breathing, which helps to deepen

your breath, at the same time oxygenating the body while focusing the mind. Simply by doing this for five minutes a day you will be both meditating and generating vital energy.

This breathing exercise (reproduced opposite with the kind permission of Oscar Ichazo), connects the Kath point— the body's center of equilibrium—with the diaphragm muscle, so that deep breathing becomes natural and effortless. You can practice it at any time, while sitting, standing, or lying down, and for as long as you like, although, ideally, find somewhere quiet first thing in the morning. You can also do it unobtrusively during moments of stress. It is an excellent natural relaxant and energy booster, helping you to feel more connected and in tune.

The diaphragm is a dome-shaped muscle attached to the bottom of the rib cage. The Kath is not an anatomical point like the navel, but is an energy point located in the lower belly, about three finger-widths below the navel. When you remember this point, you become aware of your entire body.

As you inhale, you will expand your lower belly from the *kath* point and your diaphragm muscle. This allows the lungs to fill with air from the bottom to the top. As you exhale, the belly and the diaphragm muscle relax, allowing the lungs to empty from top to bottom. Inhale and exhale through your nose.

1. Sit comfortably, in a quiet place with your spine straight.

2. Focus your attention on your Kath point.

3. Let your belly expand from the Kath point as you inhale slowly, deeply, and effortlessly. Feel your diaphragm being pulled down toward the Kath point as your lungs fill with air from the bottom to the top. On the exhale, relax both your belly and your diaphragm, emptying your lungs from top to bottom.

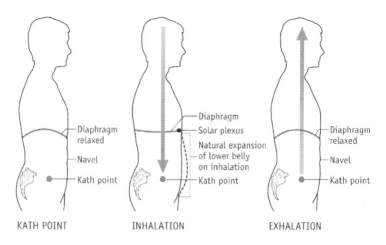

KATH POINT   INHALATION   EXHALATION

Diakath Breathing
© 2002 Oscar Ichazo. Diakath Breathing is the service mark and
Kath the trademark of Oscar Ichazo. Used by permission.

4. Repeat at your own pace.

5. Every morning, sit down in a quiet place before breakfast and practise diakath breathing for a few minutes.

6. Whenever you are stressed throughout the day, check your breathing. Practice diakath breathing for nine breaths. This is great to do before an important meeting, or when something has upset you.

Have a detoxifying massage

The body stores chemical toxins, physical tension, and negative emotions. A good massage helps to detoxify at every level by stimulating the circulation and lymphatic system, and mobilizing toxins. Regular massage is part of my ongoing strategy for detoxifying your life. Make sure you have one or two during your 9-Day Liver Detox.

Detoxify your life

Detoxification is about eliminating what is unnecessary. As you do this on the inside, by detoxifying your body, you can also detoxify your mind. For example, make a commitment to resolve an issue you have with someone. Write a comprehensive letter expressing all your negative feelings about that person's behavior or attitudes, going through every emotionally charged incident with him or her, really letting it rip, holding nothing back, telling that person that you won't accept his or her negative projections. However, don't send it! Now write a letter detailing everything you like about that person, how much you've learned from him or her, going through every incident you can recall where you felt uplifted and supported by him or her. Don't send this letter either. This simple exercise should make you clearer on what is the real issue you have with the other person, and you will feel more able to talk it through and resolve it with him or her, rather than continuing to hold on to it.

Also, why not detoxify the environment in which you live as well? Spring-clean a room in your house or workplace—perhaps your living room, bedroom, study, or office. Go through each drawer and cupboard and throw away those items that you never use. If in doubt, throw it out. Now open the windows to air the room well and then clean your room thoroughly. Buy some flowers or a plant for your room and then burn some incense or aromatherapy oil.

Chapter Four

Test Your Detox Potential— Before and After

So that you can chart your own progress, it's a good idea to rate your detox potential before and after the 9-Day Liver Detox. There are two ways you can do this: with my simple Detox Check questionnaires, and with a more objective urine or blood test. The point of checking before and after is to demonstrate the difference that even a 9-Day Liver Detox can make in your life. Even if your scores on the Detox Check are largely unchanged, you at least have the satisfaction of knowing that your liver is now better able to cope with future toxins. Doing this detox even a couple of times a year will help prevent the many chronic degenerative diseases that plague modern life, such as heart disease, cancer, and diabetes.

The two ways of testing your liver are the LiverCheck and the Detoxification Capacity Profile.

The LiverCheck

The standard medical test for overall liver function measures your levels of two liver enzymes called AST and ALT. If your levels are high, it means you may have a fatty liver or a degree of liver damage. This is well worth doing, especially if you drink alcohol on a regular basis. You get a comprehensive report telling you where you are and what to do. Your doctor can also run this test. See Resources for more details.

The Detoxification Capacity Profile

The Detoxification Capacity Profile involves a test kit that you order by mail. It explains exactly what to do and involves you taking a urine sample. It tests function rather than damage or disease. The advantage of the test is that it does help you fine-tune your supplement program. This is particularly helpful for people with chronic digestive problems or fatigue.

The test involves you swallowing a measured amount of caffeine, acetaminophen, and aspirin in a pill. You then collect your urine sample (the kit provides a container), and you'll get a report that looks like the one on the next page.

Looking at the profile report

As I described in chapter 1, phase I is where toxins are worked on by P450 enzymes to prepare them for phase II. This person's phase I is just within normal range but is verging on sluggish, so he or she would benefit from the vitamins and minerals that would help boost phase II detoxification (see chapter 1, page 23). Phase II is where toxins from phase I are "conjugated" to make them nontoxic. This person has extremely low plasma cysteine, which is used to make glutathione for glutathione conjugation. Consequently, you can see that glutathione conjugation is similarly below normal range. He or she would benefit from eating more onions and garlic for glutathione and more nuts and seeds for selenium (to help manufacture the glutathione enzymes), and supplementing N-acetylcysteine or glutathione (and eating berries to improve their utilization). This person's plasma sulfate

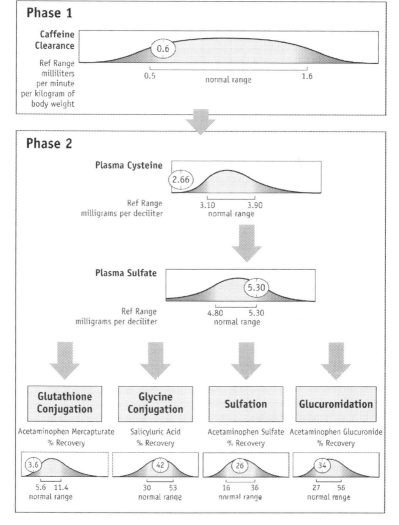

A typical Detoxification Capacity Profile report

is high, and consequently sulfation is working normally. Glycine conjugation and glucuronidation are similarly normal.

If you'd like to be guided by a test like this, see Resources to order a test kit. It also gives you the option to retest yourself to see how you've improved your liver detox function.

The Detox Check questionnaires

Below are four questionnaires that make up my Detox Check. One covers **energy**, the next **digestion**, then **detox**, and finally **aches and pains**. Each question gives you three possible scores (0, 1, or 2).

Score 0 if you never or rarely have this symptom; for example, less than once a month

Score 1 if you sometimes have this symptom; for example, more than once a month

Score 2 if you either always or frequently have this symptom; for example, at least every week

So, your worst possible score is 82. Score yourself in the "Now" column, as an average for the last month. Once you've finished your 9-Day Liver Detox, score yourself again.

QUESTIONNAIRE energy check	Now	After detox
1. Are you rarely wide awake within fifteen minutes of rising?	___	___
2. Do you need tea, coffee, a cigarette, or something sweet to get you going in the morning?	___	___
3. Do you crave chocolate, sweet foods, bread, cereal, or pasta?	___	___

4. Do you add sugar to your drinks, have
   sugared drinks, or add sugared sauces,
   such as ketchup, to your food?   ____ ____

5. Do you often have energy slumps during
   the day or after meals?   ____ ____

6. Do you crave something sweet or a
   stimulant after meals?   ____ ____

7. Do you often have mood swings or
   difficulty concentrating?   ____ ____

8. Do you get dizzy or irritable if you go
   six hours without food?   ____ ____

9. Do you find you overreact to stress?   ____ ____

10. Is your energy less now than it used to be?   ____ ____

11. Do you feel too tired to exercise?   ____ ____

Your total energy score   ____ ____

QUESTIONNAIRE digestion check

	Now	After detox
1. Do you get a burning sensation or feeling of indigestion in your stomach?	____	____
2. Do you use indigestion tablets?	____	____
3. Do you often have an uncomfortable feeling of fullness in your stomach?	____	____
4. Do you find it difficult digesting fatty foods?	____	____
5. Do you often get diarrhea?	____	____
6. Do you often suffer from constipation?	____	____
7. Do you often get a bloated stomach?	____	____
8. Do you often feel nauseous?	____	____

9. Do you often belch or pass wind?   ____ ____

10. Do you fail to have a bowel movement
    at least once a day?   ____ ____

                    Your total digestion score   ____ ____

QUESTIONNAIRE detox check

After
Now   detox

1. Do you suffer from bad breath?   ____ ____

2. Do you have watery or itchy eyes;
    swollen, red, or sticky eyelids; or
    bags or dark circles under your eyes?   ____ ____

3. Do you have itchy ears, earache, ear
    infections, drainage from the ear, or
    ringing in the ears?   ____ ____

4. Do you suffer from excessive mucus,
    a stuffy nose, or sinus problems?   ____ ____

5. Do you suffer from acne, skin rashes,
    or hives?   ____ ____

6. Do you sweat a lot and have a strong
    body odor, including your feet?   ____ ____

7. Do you have a sluggish metabolism and find
    it hard to lose weight, or are you under-
    weight and find it hard to gain weight?   ____ ____

8. Do you have a bitter taste in your mouth
    or a furry tongue?   ____ ____

9. Do you easily get a hangover and feel
    considerably worse the next day after
    just a small amount of alcohol?   ____ ____

10. Does coffee leave you feeling jittery or
    unwell?   ____ ____

                    Your total detox score   ____ ____

QUESTIONNAIRE pain check

		Now	After detox
1.	Do you suffer from headaches or migraine?	____	____
2.	Do you suffer from allergies?	____	____
3.	Do you have joint or muscle aches or pains?	____	____
4.	Do you suffer from IBS (irritable bowel syndrome)?	____	____
5.	Do you suffer from hay fever?	____	____
6.	Do you suffer from rashes, itches, eczema, or dermatitis?	____	____
7.	Do you suffer from asthma or shortness of breath?	____	____
8.	Do you suffer from colitis, diverticulitis, or Crohn's disease?	____	____
9.	Do you suffer from other aches or pains?	____	____
10.	Do you use painkillers most weeks?	____	____
	Your total pain score	____	____

Total Score

Now add up your total scores and fill them in below:

Energy ___ + **Digestion** ___ + **Detox** ___ + **Pain** ___ = ___

Ideally, what you want is a score of no more than 2 in any section and not more than 10 in total. Whatever your score is now, what's important is your score after your 9-Day Liver Detox.

Your total "after" score: _____

Above 30 (and decrease by one-third during detox): If your score is above 30 and decreases by a third or more during your 9-Day Liver Detox, keep going. You need to continue with these detox principles for a month.

Above 30 (without much change during detox): If your score is above 30 and doesn't change much during your 9-Day Liver Detox, have you been taking the recommended supplements? As well as continuing with the detox principles, see a nutritional therapist, who can advise you in more detail and, if necessary, run some tests to find out why you feel under par.

Between 10 and 29: If your score has decreased substantially and is between 10 and 29, well done. You are making progress and now need to integrate as many of these principles as you can into your daily life. Rescore yourself again after 90 days.

Below 10: You are in reasonably good health. Well done. You may choose to do an annual 9-Day Liver Detox—especially if this makes a big difference to how you feel—or you may wish to incorporate many of these principles into your daily life.

In chapter 7, I explain how to maintain your health improvements and detox for life.

PART TWO

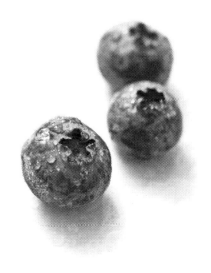

Chapter Five

Start Detoxing Now!

Your 9-Day Liver Detox is designed to be followed over two weekends, with one whole week in between. You really need the full nine days for the detox improvement to start showing up in feelings of well-being and the lessening of symptoms. The idea of the two weekends sandwiched around a full week is that it will make life as easy for you as possible in terms of shopping, preparing, and implementing the diet if you are working full-time. This gives you some time to get used to the new way of eating without the pressures and time constraints of work. If this isn't convenient, however, feel free to start whenever it suits you.

Fiona and I are going to tell you exactly what to do, down to providing your exact shopping list. The first thing you need to do is set the date—as soon as possible. Remember: Tomorrow is the most special day. Why? Because everything always happens tomorrow! So, get your diary out now and make a date. It's important to pick a week and weekends where you won't be under pressure to drink or eat vast amounts of food. It's even better if you can pick a week when you are in an environment that supports your transformation to a new you.

You will need the following for your detox, and these are itemized later in this chapter:

Food You will find complete shopping lists to see you through the detox period (see pages 98–108).

Supplements See chapter 3 for a full explanation of the supplements I suggest you take and page 110 for a chart listing when to take them.

Good-quality water In chapter 3, I explained how important it is to drink plenty of water, either bottled or filtered. On page 57, we list the requirements for your detox, as a reminder while you gather everything together in preparation.

You will also need to be clear about the rules, because following them will give you the best transformation. On pages 90–92 is a complete list of what you'll be eating and avoiding, which incorporates all the points from chapters 2 and 3.

We have given you an exact 9-Day Menu Plan, with details of all the recipes. Alternatively, you could create your own plan based on foods from the "included" list on pages 91–92. However, if you choose your own foods from the "included" list, you also need to ensure that you follow my Six Golden Liver Detox Rules listed in the box on page 89.

Following our 9-Day Menu Plan is easier than doing it yourself, because we have integrated all of the golden rules into the daily menus. Take a look now at pages 93–98 so that you have a sense of what the menus look like.

You'll notice that most of the instructions are obvious, but some link through to precise recipes when there's something you have to make. The 9-Day Menu Plan is followed by your shopping list. You need to go shopping twice during your detox—on Day 1 (Saturday), or the day before, and on Day 5 (Wednesday).

That's it. The following pages give you everything you need to know:

The Six Golden Liver Detox Rules

1. Drink eight glasses of water or fluid every day.
2. Have a tablespoon of ground seeds every day.
3. Have a serving of our Super Greens Mix every day.
4. Have a serving of cruciferous vegetables (broccoli, brussels sprouts, cabbage, cauliflower, or kale) every day.
5. Have a garlic clove, a small onion, a shallot, or four green onions every day for their sulfur content.
6. Have one of our superfood juices or smoothies every day.

What to avoid and what to eat

In chapters 2 and 3, we listed the Five Habits to Break and the Five Habits to Make. Here is a reminder of those foods for you to see at a glance.

Foods to avoid

Avoid all the following foods and drinks, as explained in chapter 2.

Wheat. You will have to avoid bread made from wheat and all commercially made cakes, biscuits, pastries, and pasta made from wheat. Also, check the labels of all other commercially made foods to ensure that no wheat is included. Instead, buy nonwheat (and preferably gluten-free) alternatives or make your own from nongluten flour (available in natural foods stores and good supermarkets). (See pages 33–38 for a full explanation of the problems with wheat on a detox.)

Dairy. You will have to avoid milk from any animal source, cheese, cream, butter, ice cream, yogurt, probiotic drinks such as Activia and kefir, and food with milk solids, whey, or casein on the label. Instead, buy rice, almond, coconut, or quinoa milk; coconut or pumpkin-seed butter, tahini, or any nut or seed butter (except peanut butter); or soy cream (or make your own with finely ground cashews and water). (See pages 38–42 for a full explanation of the problems with milk on a detox.)

Caffeine. You will have to avoid coffee, black tea, colas, diet colas, Red Bull, and other caffeinated drinks. Remember to reduce coffee to a maximum of one cup a day before starting the detox, or you could be in for a ferocious headache. If you can give up caffeine altogether before starting, that would be even better. Please do not substitute the decaffeinated versions of these drinks, as they contain potential carcinogens that also have to be detoxified. Substitute up to two cups of weak green tea, rooibos, herbal tea, or water. (See pages 42–48 for a full explanation of the problems with caffeine on a detox.)

Alcohol. Replace with mineral water or organic fruit juice. You can also try fruit smoothies as an alternative. (See pages 48–51 for a full explanation of the problems with alcohol on a detox.)

Bad fats. You will have to avoid all meat, all fried foods (including any vegetables, French fries, and potato chips), all processed foods containing hydrogenated (or partially hydrogenated) oils, commercial mayonnaise, and all margarines and spreads. Substitute with essential fats from fish (but not fried fish), eggs, olive oil, raw nuts and seeds, and nut and seed butters and oils. (But don't cook with them; if you are intending to use oil in cooking, use only olive oil.) See pages 52–54 for a full explanation of the problems with bad fats on a detox.

Essential foods

If you are not following the 9-Day Menu Plan on pages 92–98, it is important that you stick rigidly to the Five Habits to Break and the Five Habits to Make. In accordance with these, we have put together a list of absolutely essential detox foods for you to stock up on.

A large quantity of bottled water (if you do not have a water filter). Bear in mind that you could be drinking 2 quarts a day. The detox potential is enhanced if you have a mug of hot water with the juice of half a lemon twice a day, as this encourages bile flow, which helps remove toxins. So, you will also need nine lemons.

Seeds (pumpkin, sunflower, sesame, and flax). These contain the omega-3 and omega-6 essential fats to help repair damaged cell membranes. They are also rich in the minerals needed for the detoxification and antioxidant enzymes. You will need enough for one tablespoon a day.

Dark green leafy vegetables (baby spinach, watercress, basil, parsley). These vegetables are rich in vitamin C, folate, chlorophyll, and antioxidants. They are best eaten raw in a salad, as cooking destroys their vitamin content.

Cruciferous vegetables (brassicas). These include broccoli (or preferably, broccolini, because you can eat the tender stems raw), brussels sprouts, cabbage, cauliflower, kale, turnips, and kohlrabi. These contain a number of essential compounds that help support detoxification. So that you will not lose the benefits of all the vitamins, steam or lightly stir-fry only or try adding raw broccoli (or broccolini, if possible) to vegetable juices.

Onions (green onions, shallots, garlic, and especially red onions). These produce the sulfur necessary for the detoxification process and can reduce inflammation. Again, eat raw if you can!

Vegetable juice. Make juice with any of the vegetables mentioned above and experiment with adding carrots, mixed peppers, tomatoes, celery, and apples, which are all high in antioxidants. The pectin in apples helps transport toxins out of the body.

Fruit juice. Make juice with any combination of berries (especially strawberries, blueberries, and raspberries) and pomegranates for their antioxidant properties.

Protein from eggs and oily fish (salmon, trout, herring, mackerel, sardines, anchovies, and fresh tuna—but eat tuna only once during the nine days, as it contains heavy metals). Eggs are the purest form of protein, and they also contain sulfur for detoxification, whereas oily fish are rich in omega-3 essential fats. Have the eggs boiled to avoid adding any fats during cooking.

Your 9-Day Menu Plan

The following menu plan is specifically designed with your new goals in mind—to make it easy to stick to your new habits (see chapter 3) and to help you break the old habits (see chapter 2). The dishes are jam-packed with superfoods, antioxidants, and water to meet your daily goals, as well as being free from caffeine, alcohol, bad fats, wheat, and milk. You can follow our menu plan here or come up with your own, following our guidelines (outlined on page 89). Unless an exact quantity is specified in the menu, feel free to eat as much of the premitted foods as you like. We have included some repeated recipes to allow you to cook in quantity and save time.

Day 1 (Saturday)

Breakfast: Superfood Muesli with Essential Seed Mix

Morning snack: Two plums plus a small handful of almonds

Lunch: Superboost Sesame Salad with a serving of Super Greens Mix

Afternoon snack: Olives and your daily smoothie or juice

Supper: Fennel and Mixed Rice Pilaf with a large tossed salad

Drinks: One fresh juice or smoothie (ideally, have a juice containing carrot and a juice containing berries or watermelon on alternate days if you haven't eaten these foods already during the day), plus unlimited water, herbal teas, and coffee alternatives

Day 2 (Sunday)

Breakfast: Superfruit and Seed Salad including Essential Seed Mix

Morning snack: Hummus with crudités

Lunch: Trout en Papillote with Roasted Vegetables followed by Fruit Burst Frozen Yogurt

Afternoon snack: Pomegranate or grapefruit

Supper: Patrick's Primordial Soup with a serving of Super Greens Mix stirred in

Drinks: One fresh juice or smoothie (ideally, have a juice containing carrot and a juice containing berries or watermelon on alternate days if you haven't eaten these foods already during the day), plus unlimited water, herbal teas, and coffee alternatives

At the end of Day 2

You may now be experiencing a few withdrawal symptoms from all the toxins you were consuming earlier: headache, nausea, and possibly light-headedness. These are nothing to worry about. Just remember, there is a direct correlation between the withdrawal symptoms and the amount of toxins previously consumed.

Day 3 (Monday)

Breakfast: Cinnamon Fruit Oatmeal including Essential Seed Mix

Morning snack: Avocado with lemon juice

Lunch: Skin-Defense Dip with arugula on pumpernickel-style rye bread

Afternoon snack: Corn on the Cob, plus your daily smoothie or juice

Supper: Age-Defying Carrot and Lentil Soup (make a double batch for lunch tomorrow) with a serving of Super Greens Mix stirred in

Drinks: One fresh juice or smoothie (ideally, have a juice containing carrot and a juice containing berries or watermelon on alternate days if you haven't eaten these foods already during the day), plus unlimited water, herbal teas, and coffee alternatives

Day 4 (Tuesday)

Breakfast: Berry Breakfast Smoothie including Essential Seed Mix

Morning snack: Hummus with crudités

Lunch: Age-Defying Carrot and Lentil Soup (left over from yesterday)

Afternoon snack: Apple plus a small handful of walnuts

Supper: Rice with Super Greens Pesto

Drinks: One fresh juice or smoothie (ideally, have a juice containing carrot and a juice containing berries or watermelon on alternate days if you haven't eaten these foods already during the day), plus unlimited water, herbal teas, and coffee alternatives

At the end of Day 4

By now, I would expect all the withdrawal symptoms to have passed, and you will be settling into the new routine of healthy eating. Remember, you never have to go hungry. Eat as much as you like of all the permitted foods.

Day 5 (Wednesday)

Breakfast: Superfruit and Seed Salad including Essential Seed Mix

Morning snack: Pear with a small handful of pecans

Lunch: Superfood Sandwich for Beautiful Skin, including Super Greens Mix

Afternoon snack: Guacamole with crudités

Supper: Leek, Cannellini, and Potato Soup (double up on the quantities for lunch tomorrow)

Drinks: One fresh juice or smoothie (ideally, have a juice containing carrot and a juice containing berries or watermelon on alternate days if you haven't eaten these foods already during the day), plus unlimited water, herbal teas and coffee alternatives

Day 6 (Thursday)

Breakfast: Superfood Muesli including Essential Seed Mix

Morning snack: Toasted pumpkin and sunflower seeds, plus a piece of fruit, if you like

Lunch: Leek, Cannellini, and Potato Soup (left over from yesterday) with a serving of Super Greens Mix stirred in

Afternoon snack: Hummus with crudités

Supper: Cleansing Bean and Artichoke Salad

Drinks: One fresh juice or smoothie (ideally, have a juice containing carrot and a juice containing berries or watermelon on alternate days if you haven't eaten these foods already during the day), plus unlimited water, herbal teas, and coffee alternatives

At the end of Day 6

Well done for sticking to the healthy-eating regime this far. You have now been on the detox diet for almost a week, and I would expect some of the benefits have become apparent: increased energy, feeling more refreshed on waking, and fewer energy dips during the day.

Day 7 (Friday)

Breakfast: Cinnamon Fruit Oatmeal with a serving of Essential Seed Mix

Morning snack: Nectarine (or other seasonal fruit) with a small handful of cashews

Lunch: Superboost Sesame Salad with a serving of Super Greens Mix

Afternoon snack: Olives, plus a piece of fruit, if you like

Supper: Baked Sweet Potatoes with Bean Stew

Drinks: One fresh juice or smoothie (ideally, have a juice containing carrot and a juice containing berries or watermelon on alternate days if you haven't eaten these foods already during the day), plus unlimited water, herbal teas, and coffee alternatives

Day 8 (Saturday)

Breakfast: Toast and Nut Butter

Morning snack: Apple, plus a small handful of cashews

Lunch: Raw Summer Soup (or one of the hot soups, if out of season) with a serving of Super Greens Mix stirred in

Afternoon snack: Raw baby corn with hummus

Supper: Mushroom and Pine Nut–Stuffed Peppers with a large tossed salad

Drinks: One fresh juice or smoothie (ideally, have a juice containing carrot and a juice containing berries or watermelon on alternate days if you haven't eaten these foods already during the day), plus unlimited water, herbal teas, and coffee alternatives

Day 9 (Sunday)

Breakfast: Berry Breakfast Smoothie including Essential Seed Mix

Morning snack: Toasted Pumpkin Seeds

Lunch: Salmon with French Green Lentils followed by Detox Pear and Blueberry Crumble

Afternoon snack: Olives, plus your daily smoothie or juice

Supper: Superfood Salad of Quinoa with Roasted Vegetables, including Super Greens Mix

Drinks: One fresh juice or smoothie (ideally, have a juice containing carrot and a juice containing berries or watermelon on alternate days if you haven't eaten these foods already during the day), plus unlimited water, herbal teas, and coffee alternatives

At the end of Day 9

Congratulations! You have now completed my 9-Day Liver Detox. I hope you are now seeing and feeling the benefits of all the health and energy improvements. But even if they are not all that you had hoped for, you can at least know that you have done a significant amount to ward off the many degenerative diseases that can result from an overloaded liver.

That having been said, please do not relapse into all your old habits now, however comfortable. How about making one of my detox diet changes permanent, such as eating broccoli several times a week or reducing drinking coffee by one cup per day and substituting an herbal tea. Then, when you come to repeat my 9-Day Liver Detox, it will be all the easier for you.

Your shopping lists

It is worth stocking up on the following foods to help you follow the nine-day plan. This will also save extra trips to the supermarket during the week when temptation might lead you to the chocolate aisle! You can find all the items in good supermarkets and natural foods stores.

Shopping list for Day 1

(for example, Saturday) or the day before
Read through the recipes in chapter 6 before making your list in case you want to make any adjustments to suit your personal

preferences, but remember to stick with healthy alternatives as explained in chapter 3 and in this chapter.

VEGETABLES

2 garlic bulbs

Bag of red onions

Bag of white onions

Bag of baby spinach

Bunch of watercress

Mixed salad greens

Bunch of basil

Bunch of celery

1 fennel bulb

Large bag of carrots

Bag of cremini mushrooms, about 6 ounces

1 globe eggplant

1 ear of corn

2 avocados

6 medium or 3 large sweet potatoes

Bunch of green onions

2 zucchini

2 beets

Small piece of fresh ginger

Two or three cruciferous vegetables, such as broccoli (or, preferably, broccolini), brussels sprouts, cabbage, cauliflower, or kale

Bag of alfalfa sprouts

Bunch of fresh flat-leaf parsley

Bunch of fresh basil

FRUIT

2 pomegranates

Bag of lemons

1 pink grapefruit

A few bananas (not too ripe)

1 watermelon

Mango (optional)

Kiwifruit (optional)

2 baskets of blueberries, or 1 basket of blueberries and
1 basket of other berries such as raspberries

Cherries

3 red bell peppers

2 plums

Bag of apples

REFRIGERATOR

Flaxseeds

1 bag of pumpkin seeds, about 8 ounces

1 bag of sesame seeds, about 8 ounces

1 bag of sunflower seeds, about 8 ounces

1 bag of sliced almonds, about 8 ounces

2 rainbow trout, filleted (if serving two people,
otherwise buy 1)

Large container of soy yogurt (choose an organic brand
with no added sugar)

2 containers hummus

FREEZER

1 bag, about 1 pound, frozen mixed berries

PANTRY

Large bag of old-fashioned rolled oats

Small bag of quick-cooking rolled oats

Bag of brown rice (preferably basmati)

Small bag of mixed rice (such as wild rice, brown basmati rice, and red rice)

Bag of quinoa

Small bag of pearl barley

1 box rice cakes

Bags of nuts (such as walnuts, pine nuts, almonds, hazelnuts, pecans, cashews)

Bag of ground almonds (almond meal)

Bag of dried coconut flakes

Oil-packed sun-dried tomatoes (optional)

1 jar nut butter

1 jar green olives

1 jar kalamata olives

2 jars marinated artichoke hearts

2 cans pinto, red, cannellini, or Great Northern beans

1 can green lentils

1 can tomatoes

1 can mixed beans

2 cans chickpeas

Bag of French green lentils (dried)

Bag of red lentils (dried)

Natural mineral water (if you don't have a water filter)

Ground cinnamon

Ground turmeric

Black peppercorns

1 container low-sodium vegetable broth powder

Small bottle of coconut oil or olive oil

Small bottle of cold-pressed extra-virgin olive oil, or flaxseed or hempseed oil

Small bottle of toasted sesame oil

(Note: If you are worried about the initial outlay, stick to olive oil rather than the more expensive flaxseed or hempseed oil, and bear in mind that all of these ingredients can be easily used up after the detox is finished.)

Can of coconut milk

Carton of rice milk (optional)

Can of tomato paste

Bag of xylitol (a safe sugar alternative sourced from plants, available in good supermarkets and natural foods stores)

Caffeine-free drink alternatives (see below)

Pumpernickel-style rye bread

For smoothies: You will also need your chosen fruits and vegetables for juices and smoothies (see pages 153–54).

Seeds and green leafy vegetables and herbs: You will need enough for your daily servings of Essential Seed Mix and the Super Greens Mix respectively (see pages 116–17 and page 129). You may need to stock up on these through the week, especially the fresh greens, once you have decided which combinations you prefer.

DRINKS

Don't forget to try some of the following caffeine-free alternatives to tea and coffee.

Herbal and fruit teas such as peppermint, chamomile, lemon, and ginger.

Rooibos (red bush) tea, a South African leaf tea, is naturally caffeine free and very popular with black tea fans, as although it does not taste the same, it has a similarly strong flavor and can be drunk with or without milk. On the 9-Day Liver Detox, substitute soy or rice milk for cow's milk.

Dandelion coffee is a liver-friendly substitute for coffee, but don't expect it to taste like the real thing!

Shopping list for Day 5
(for example, Wednesday)
Check to see whether you need to restock items such as nuts and seeds that you are eating every day.

VEGETABLES

Bunch of celery

Bag of baby spinach

Bunch of watercress

Mixed salad greens

Bag of alfalfa sprouts

More fresh basil and parsley if your supplies
    need replenishing

Bunch of cilantro

Small bag or a handful of new potatoes

Two or three cruciferous vegetables, such as broccoli
    (or, preferably, broccolini), brussels sprouts, cabbage,
    cauliflower, or kale

1 large sweet potato, or 2 small to medium ones, plus another small one

1 ear of corn

A few baby corn cobs

4 large red bell peppers

4 shallots (optional)

Bag of cremini mushrooms, about 6 ounces

Bunch of green onions

1 avocado

1 small cucumber

4 large leeks

1 small zucchini

2 pounds cherry tomatoes

FRUIT

Small bunch of bananas (not too ripe)

Several baskets of blueberries (buy a couple now and then; buy more when you need them, to avoid waste)

1 pomegranate

3 pears

1 nectarine (or other seasonal fruit)

Bag of apples

REFRIGERATOR

3 salmon fillets, preferably wild (if serving two people; otherwise buy 2)

Large container of hummus

Container of guacamole (or an extra avocado to make your own)

You will also need to replenish your supplies of fruit and vegetables for juices and smoothies to see you through the remainder of the plan, as well as rice cakes, lemons, carrots, onions, and garlic, if you have used up your supplies from earlier in the week.

General shopping list

If you are not following the 9-Day Menu Plan on pages 92–98, we have put together a more general list of foods that are used in the recipes, for you to stock up on.

Purchase an assortment of fruit and vegetables according to your likes and what is in season or available. Here are some suggestions.

VEGETABLES

> Two or three cruciferous vegetables, such as broccoli (or, preferably, broccolini), brussels sprouts, cabbage, cauliflower, or kale
>
> Avocados
>
> Baby corn
>
> Baby spinach
>
> Basil
>
> Carrots
>
> Celery
>
> Cilantro
>
> Corn on the cob
>
> Eggplant
>
> Flat-leaf parsley
>
> Ginger
>
> Garlic

Leeks

Lettuce or mixed salad greens

Mixed bell peppers

Mushrooms

Pumpkin or squash

Red onions

Sweet potatoes

Tomatoes

Watercress

White onions

Zucchini

FRUIT

Apples

Bananas

Berries (for example, blueberries, strawberries, and raspberries)

Grapes

Kiwifruit

Lemons

Mangos

Oranges

Pears

Pink grapefruit

Pomegranate

Watermelon

REFRIGERATOR

Hummus

Guacamole (if not making your own)

Soy yogurt (choose an organic brand with no added sugar)

Sunflower, pumpkin, and sesame seeds

Flaxseeds

Salmon fillets

Trout fillets

Omega-rich seed-oil blend

FREEZER

Peas

Mixed berries

PANTRY

Unsalted nut butter

Old-fashioned rolled oats

Ground almonds (almond meal)

Tahini (sesame paste)

Xylitol (a safe sugar alternative sourced from plants, available in good supermarkets and natural foods stores)

Coconut oil or olive oil for cooking

Extra-virgin olive oil

Toasted sesame oil

Olives

Canned mixed beans

Canned or dried chickpeas

Canned or dried pinto, red, cannellini, or Great Northern beans

Dried French green lentils

Quinoa

Ground ginger

Ground cinnamon

Ground turmeric

Dried herbes de Provence or mixed dried herbs

Marinated artichoke hearts

Canned coconut milk

Rice milk

Pine nuts

Mixed nuts

Low-sodium vegetable broth powder

Tomato paste

Natural mineral water (if you don't have a water filter)

Preparing for the Six Golden Liver Detox Rules

1. Drink eight glasses of water or fluid every day

This is the equivalent of about 3 pints (48 fluid ounces) water, and can be drunk cold or hot, as in noncaffeine teas. Add half a lemon squeezed into a mug of hot water twice a day. Choose either filtered water or bottled natural mineral water.

2. Have a tablespoon of ground seeds every day

Seeds are incredibly rich in essential fats, minerals, vitamin E, protein, and fiber. Make up our Essential Seed Mix (see page 116) to add to your cereal each day.

3. Have a serving of our Super Greens Mix every day

Each day, make a Super Greens Mix (see page 129) using a handful each of baby spinach leaves, watercress, parsley, and basil, with variations, such as sun-dried tomatoes, artichoke hearts, pine nuts, pumpkin seeds, and avocado.

4. Have a serving of cruciferous vegetables

Eat a serving of broccoli (or, preferably, broccolini), brussels sprouts, cabbage, cauliflower, or kale every day. These are ideally eaten raw or can be lightly steamed or stir-fried in a small amount of oil, or try steam-frying, below.

Steam-Frying

Add about 2 tablespoons liquid (such as water, vegetable stock, or a watered-down sauce) to a wok or large skillet—use one with a lid. When the liquid is boiling, add your vegetables and stir-fry for about 1 minute, then cover and cook for 2 minutes. Turn down the heat and steam until the vegetables are crisp-tender—you can always add a splash more water if the pan dries out.

5. Have a garlic clove, a small onion or shallot, or 4 green onions every day

Sulfur up your diet with these health-giving vegetables each day. Eat them raw if possible.

6. Have one of our superfood juices or smoothies every day

Choose from our menu of delicious superfood juices and smoothies, which include refreshing and healthy fruits such as berries, watermelon, and citrus fruits (see pages 155–59).

Your liver detox supplement support program

The following chart gives you the supplements to take during your 9-Day Liver Detox to get the best results. Remember to take detox supplements every day.

	DOSAGE		
	Breakfast	Lunch	Dinner
During the 9-Day Liver Detox			
Digestive enzymes/ probiotics/glutamine	1	1	1
Glutamine powder			1 tsp at bedtime
Antioxidant/liver-support formula	1	1	
Every day			
High-potency multivitamin	1	1	
Vitamin C	1	1	
Essential fats (EPA, DHA, and GLA)	1		

Troubleshooting

Most people will have no trouble at all on this diet and will feel great by the end. Just occasionally, though, you might feel a bit rough at the beginning. Here is what might happen and what to do about it.

Withdrawal symptoms

I have already talked about the need to reduce coffee to a maximum of one cup a day before starting the detox to minimize the risk of headaches. This is because caffeine is an addictive substance and you will be going through withdrawal. The same may also be true of any food you have given up (such as wheat and dairy) to which you are allergic or sensitive. You may not just have a headache, you may feel weak and nauseous as well, and you may find yourself craving the food (or caffeine) you have given up.

This is a very clear indication that you are indeed sensitive to these foods, and I would recommend that you cut them out of your diet completely for three months and then reintroduce them one at a time and very slowly. Unfortunately, there is nothing to be done about these symptoms except to drink even more water and to rest. They should pass in twenty-four to thirty-six hours.

Cravings can be combated to some extent by having a substitute food. For example, if you are craving dairy foods, nibble on mixed seeds or dip some bread into flaxseed oil; this will provide you with an alternative fat but one that will only do you good. Sugar cravings can be reduced by taking a chromium supplement (200 mcg of chromium) or having a teaspoon of glutamine powder.

Coated tongue, bad breath, and body odor

Believe it or not, a coated tongue, bad breath, or body odor is a good sign, demonstrating that your body really is detoxing. They will pass after a few days.

Meanwhile, shower regularly but do not use soap, shower gel, or deodorant unless they come from a natural foods store and are free of toxic chemicals and heavy metals (deodorants usually contain aluminum). Clean your teeth regularly but gently (don't allow your gums to bleed), preferably with toothpaste that, similarly, does not contain fluoride or other toxic chemicals. Do not use mouthwash. Keep drinking water to encourage the toxins to leave your body in urine rather than sweat and saliva.

Constipation or diarrhea

You are unlikely to suffer from constipation because you will be eating so much more fiber and drinking so many more fluids. If it occurs, it will just be the body's way of adjusting to your new eating habits. Don't take any laxatives. It will pass quickly.

Diarrhea is more common and is just the result of the additional fiber combined with the body adjusting to not having the usual constipating proteins and refined carbohydrates. However, you lose additional fluids when you have diarrhea, so be sure to drink even more water. The diarrhea should pass in a couple of days, but if it does not, then leave out all nuts and seeds and cut out vitamin C supplements until you pass normally formed stools, then resume.

Be aware that the number of bowel movements in a day will almost certainly increase. This is a good development and indicates that you are not reabsorbing toxins in your intestine. A mucus-coated stool will indicate that you are actually detoxing from the colon as well. Two to three bowel movements a day would be a very healthy number on this detox diet.

Other symptoms

Detoxification can also induce nausea, aches and pains, fatigue, and nasal discharge. This is because toxins are being released into the bloodstream at a faster rate than the liver can detoxify them. These symptoms will pass after a couple of days.

The best remedy is to go for a sauna or use a steam room. This forces the toxins out of the bloodstream and into the skin, where they are released as sweat, bypassing the log-jammed liver. The best regimen is to sweat for ten to fifteen minutes, then to have a cold shower, then go back into the sauna or steam room. Keep this up for as long as you feel comfortable, but stop if you feel at all faint or dizzy. Drink even more water, as you will be losing a lot in sweat. If you can't cope with the heat, then go for a run to work up a sweat.

Eating some of the foods we have listed in this chapter may be new to you, but when you look through the collection of tasty liver detox recipes that Fiona has prepared for you in the following chapter we are sure you will feel motivated and enthusiastic about getting started on your 9-Day Liver Detox. She also explains how to prepare our basic superfoods: the Essential Seed Mix (page 116) and Super Greens Mix (page 119).

Chapter Six

Your 9-Day Liver Detox Recipes

I feel particularly qualified to write the recipes for this book not only because I am a nutritionist and cook but also because I have recently undergone a detox myself. People always expect nutritionists to be positively radiating good health and vitality, but often the very reason that we turned to nutrition in the first place is because of our own health problems. I followed the detox rules here in order to sort out some skin problems while I was developing these recipes, and am happy to report great results! This has given me firsthand experience of what it is like to cut out favorite foods, not to mention an insight into the need for appetizing recipes to boost morale when you are not feeling your best or are craving "off-limits" foods. The result, I hope, is a collection of recipes that are appetizing and interesting and are positively packed with nutrients to cleanse your liver and boost your health.

There is no doubt about it, detoxing is hard work. It is hard work for your body, as your liver will be straining to keep up with pressure to eliminate waste and toxins, and it is hard work physically for you: Mealtimes need planning and preparation. You cannot simply grab a sandwich or a plate of pasta, or boost flagging energy levels with a cup of coffee. We do understand that what we are asking you to do is hard, so we have taken particular care to come up with appetizing, filling meals that should help to keep your spirits high during the nine-day plan.

—Fiona McDonald Joyce

Breakfast

It is important to start the day with a nutritious meal to kick-start your metabolism and provide you with energy at the best of times, but particularly so during a detox. Your liver function peaks between 2 a.m. and 4 a.m., so by the time you wake your body has already been at work for hours. You therefore need to refuel, and in particular get some protein inside you to allow the liver's detoxification process to continue. For those people who "don't do breakfast," a smoothie or fresh juice is a refreshing and energizing start to the day. You may also wish to have a glass of hot water with the freshly squeezed juice of half a lemon before eating in the morning. Lemons are very rich in vitamin C—much more so than their more acclaimed cousin the orange—and make a very cleansing drink to prepare your body for digestion and detoxification. You can add a couple of slices of fresh ginger to the mug for a more warming flavor if you like.

Why add the Essential Seed Mix?

Seeds are a vital part of your diet and are particularly helpful during a detox. They contain essential fats to keep your hormones in balance and your skin looking great, as well as minerals such as zinc to keep your immune system functioning and your blood sugar under control, and magnesium to give your thyroid a boost. They also provide protein, which your liver needs each day to detox efficiently and prevent the toxins you are releasing from being reabsorbed by the body. Our Essential Seed Mix is an easy way to include the recommended tablespoon of seeds in your diet at breakfast each day. Simply add a tablespoon of the ground seed mix to breakfast cereal, fruit salad, or smoothies.

Essential Seed Mix

Fill a glass jar with a lid halfway with flaxseeds (rich in omega-3) and top it off with a mixture of sesame, sunflower, and pumpkin seeds (rich in omega-6).

Keep the jar sealed and in the fridge to minimize damage from light, heat, and oxygen.

Put a handful of the seed mix in a coffee or spice grinder (see Detox Tip, opposite), grind it up, and add a tablespoon to your cereal. Store the remainder in the fridge and use over the next few days.

To save time, you could grind up to a week's worth of seeds, but make sure you store them away from heat, light, and air to prevent the delicate essential fats from oxidizing.

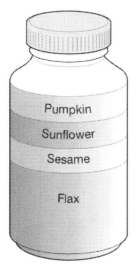

The proportions of seeds in the Essential Seed Mix

Detox Tip

Grinding the seeds makes the nutrients in them available to the body; otherwise, tiny seeds like flaxseeds or sesame seeds are too small to be digested. If you don't have time to grind seeds you could simply sprinkle larger seeds such as pumpkin and sunflower seeds straight onto your food, together with precracked or ground flaxseeds, which you can buy from supermarkets (in the natural foods aisle) and natural foods stores. Buy ones stored in foil or other lightproof packaging, however, to ensure that the fats are protected from oxidation before you get them home and into the fridge.

Superfood Muesli   SERVES 1

This thick, soaked muesli is delicious and particularly nutritious, as all the ingredients are raw, maximizing the vitamin, enzyme, and antioxidant content. Apples contain the phytonutrient quercetin, which is a natural anti-inflammatory that helps with allergies, asthma, eczema, and arthritis. Oats are a fiber-rich, low-glycemic-load carbohydrate; that is, they release their energy very slowly to keep you feeling fuller for longer; they also contain the amino acid tryptophan, which the brain converts into the "feel-good" neurotransmitter serotonin.

$1/2$ cup old-fashioned rolled oats
1 tablespoon ground almonds or dried flaked coconut
1 tablespoon Essential Seed Mix (page 116)
$1/2$ small apple, grated
1 tablespoon fresh berries (such as raspberries or blueberries)
$1/2$ teaspoon ground cinnamon, or to taste (optional)

Place all the ingredients in a bowl and cover with double the amount of boiling water. Stir and leave to thicken for a couple of minutes until the oats have soaked up the water and become soft and plump.

Cinnamon Fruit Oatmeal SERVES 1

Oats are full of soluble fiber for healthy digestion and release their energy very slowly to keep you filled up. Cinnamon not only adds a wonderfully warming flavor, but it is also a valuable nutrient, helping the body regulate blood sugar levels. Ground ginger can be used instead of the cinnamon or in addition, if you prefer.

$^1/_2$ cup old-fashioned rolled oats
$^1/_2$ to 1 teaspoon ground cinnamon, or to taste
1 tablespoon Essential Seed Mix (page 116)
Chopped or grated fruit or whole berries (see Cook's Tip)

Place the oats in a saucepan and cover with water. Bring to a boil, then gently simmer, stirring, until the cereal thickens and the oats soften.

Stir the cinnamon, seed mix, and fruit into the oatmeal, or simply scatter on top of the oatmeal in a bowl.

Cook's Tip

Chop or coarsely grate $^1/_2$ apple, or chop up a pear or a couple of plums or apricots, or simply toss some berries into the cereal and let them soften in the heat so that they burst and release their sweet juice.

Toast and Nut Butter   SERVES 1

Here we use pumpernickel-style rye bread, as it contains less gluten than wheat, making it much easier to digest. Plus, wholegrain rye is a good source of prebiotics, feeding the good bacteria in your gut. Spread it with nut or seed butter (you can get a whole range of different nut and seed butters in natural foods stores) to add some protein to help fuel your liver's detoxification pathways, as well as to fill you up.

1 thin slice pumpernickel-style rye bread
1 tablespoon (or enough to spread on each slice) nut or seed butter (almond and hazelnut are particularly good)

Toast the bread, then spread the nut butter on each slice. There is enough natural oil in nuts and seeds for you not to miss regular butter—honestly.

Superfruit and Seed Salad   SERVES 1

If going on a detox makes you feel instantly deprived as you give up your usual morning cappuccino or croissant, think about the money you will be saving and splurge instead on some tropical fruit or fresh berries to enliven breakfast. Not only do their bright, vibrant colors look wonderful, they are also packed with phytonutrients like flavonoids to really kick-start your immune system. Apply the Rainbow Rule (opposite) and try to get as many different colors into your bowl as possible, as each color indicates a different type of plant nutrient.

Seeds of ¹/₂ pomegranate
Watermelon chunks (leave the seeds in as
   they are rich in vitamin E)
2 handfuls fresh blueberries
Or
Mango slices
Banana slices
Fresh strawberries
Sliced kiwifruit

1 tablespoon Essential Seed Mix (page 116)
A good squeeze of fresh lemon juice

Mix the fruits in a bowl with the seed mix and gently stir in the
lemon juice. (Lemon juice not only adds a pleasing tartness to
complement the sweet fruit, but also the vitamin C prevents
the cut fruit from oxidizing and turning brown and the liquid
helps loosen the texture of the dry seeds.)

The Rainbow Rule

Aim to eat as many different colors of fruits and vegetables as
possible, as each color denotes a particular health benefit. For
example, yellow and orange plants such as squash, peppers,
and sweet potatoes are rich in the antioxidant vitamin beta-
carotene, which has valuable antiaging properties, whereas the
rich pinks, purples, and blues in berries are high in free-radical-
scavenging flavonoids, which again will help you hold back
the years. In your superfruit salad, try unpeeled apples, pears,
pluots, apricots, peaches, nectarines, plums, oranges, tangerines, kiwifruit, or pomegranate to vary the colors. By eating
the fruit raw, you benefit from all of the nutrient content, from
vitamins and minerals to phytonutrients and enzymes. Plus,
fruit is packed with fiber and water, both of which will keep your
digestive system working and help reduce bloating.

Berry Breakfast Smoothie   SERVES 1

If you don't have the time or inclination for breakfast, then go for a smoothie. You can drink it on the run, and it is packed with all the nutrients you need: carbohydrates, vitamins, and minerals from the fruit, and essential fats and protein from the seeds. This can count as your breakfast or as your daily juice or smoothie (according to our Six Golden Liver Detox Rules on page 89), but not as both. Blueberries are particularly rich in immune- and liver-boosting flavonoids, but you can vary the fruit used. Also, after your detox, when you can eat dairy products again, try thickening the smoothie with live-culture natural yogurt to add extra protein and beneficial probiotic bacteria.

> 1 small or $1/2$ medium banana, not too ripe
> 2 teaspoons Essential Seed Mix (page 116)
> 1 cup fresh blueberries or other berries
> Juice of $1/2$ lemon
> Enough pure fruit juice (orange works well) or unsweetened
>   rice milk (or other nondairy milk; see Detox Tip, below)
>   or waterto give an easy-to-drink consistency (or leave
>   thick and eat with a spoon)

Using a blender, puree all the ingredients together until smooth.

Detox Tip

Other nondairy milks to try are quinoa, almond, oat, soy, or coconut milk.

Snacks

Here are some quick snack ideas to keep your energy levels balanced and your liver functioning efficiently. They are all super quick to make, and there are lots of easy, convenient options such as fruit and nuts to keep in your drawer at work or in your bag if you are out and about.

Fruit

It's not original, but fruit is about as fast as food gets and, of course, it is incredibly good for you. Again, think beyond the usual apple or orange (although these are still nutrient-packed choices) to get some different colors and phytonutrients into your diet. You could pick at a basket of berries, or have fresh apricots, a slice of melon, a pink grapefruit, or perhaps kiwi, mango, or red grapes rather than green. If you are the kind of person who normally peels your apple or pear, don't—much of the goodness is stored in the skin. Many fruit seeds are good for you as well, such as those in grapes (go for seeded rather than the more expensive seedless varieties), and watermelon, which has seeds rich in the skin-friendly antioxidant vitamin E. Apple seeds, however, do contain a toxin and are best not eaten.

Have a small handful (around a tablespoon) of nuts or seeds with your fruit to provide extra protein, which will fill you up for longer and boost the detoxification process.

Nuts and seeds

Nibble on a small handful (around a tablespoon) of unsalted, unroasted nuts or seeds (such as pecans, almonds, walnuts, Brazil nuts, hazelnuts, pumpkin seeds, or sunflower seeds, or a mixture of your favorites). Eating nuts or seeds with fruit helps to keep blood sugar even, as the protein slows down the release of sugar from the fruit into the bloodstream. They are also packed with minerals such as zinc, which is involved in everything from your immune system to hormone balance and even libido.

Toasted pumpkin seeds

Heat a skillet before putting the pumpkin seeds into it (no oil needed) and cook for a couple of minutes, tossing the seeds in the pan occasionally, until they start to pop and turn golden.

Olives

Olives contain heart-healthy monounsaturated fats. They are also a quick and easy snack that is very filling. Look for ones stuffed with whole garlic cloves or almonds, for extra liver-boosting power. Eat a handful, or about eight olives, as a snack.

Avocado

Also rich in monounsaturated fats, avocados also contain vitamin E. Avocados act as "nutrient boosters," increasing the body's ability to absorb fat-soluble nutrients like alpha- and beta-carotene from other foods. They also provide over twenty-five nutrients, including fiber, potassium, vitamin E, B vitamins, and folic acid. A couple over the course of the nine-day plan are fine, but don't have too many, as you don't want to add too much fat to your diet. A half or a whole avocado makes a delicious snack: simply cut in half, remove the pit, and drizzle with lemon juice or enjoy it plain. You can also follow the Mexicans' example and mash avocado onto toast instead of butter. If you are eating only half, keep the pit in the remaining half, drizzle with lemon juice, wrap in plastic wrap, and keep in the fridge to prevent it from discoloring. Eat it the next day.

Hummus with crudités

Hummus is a fantastic snack and light-meal standby for when you are busy. The chickpeas in hummus provide protein, plus fiber and phytoestrogens to help keep your hormones in balance, while the garlic will replenish your sulfur levels to help your liver's detoxification capacity. Grab a container from the refrigerator aisle in the supermarket or deli and dip in crudités, such as celery, apple, cucumber, and pepper strips, or try rice cakes for a more substantial snack or light lunch. Store-bought hummus will contain a little salt, but it is still a healthy and extremely convenient choice during a detox, and makes for a perfect detox snack or lunch on the go. Stir in a dollop of Super Greens Mix (page 129) to make it extra healthy.

Guacamole

If you have a little more time, you can make this delicious, very refreshing avocado dip and serve it with crudités. Don't just stick to the usual carrot, celery, and cucumber crudités; try sugar snap peas, baby corn, cabbage, radishes, green onions, celery root, bell peppers, cherry tomatoes, and fennel.

1 ripe avocado
Juice of $^1/_4$ lemon
$^1/_2$ clove garlic, crushed
$^1/_4$ small red onion, finely diced
3 cherry tomatoes, finely diced
1 tablespoon chopped fresh cilantro or flat-leaf parsley,
    or a combination of both (optional)
1 tablespoon extra-virgin olive oil or omega-rich seed oil
    such as flaxseed, hempseed, or pumpkin-seed oil
    (optional)
Freshly ground pepper

Cut the avocado in half lengthwise and remove the pit.

Scrape the flesh out of the shell into a bowl and quickly mash with the remaining ingredients, then taste to check the seasoning. (Keep any leftovers covered in the fridge for up to 2 days.)

Corn on the Cob SERVES 1

This is a very filling snack, and the bright yellow corn kernels are packed with beta-carotene, an essential antioxidant for the skin. Most people slather corn on the cob with butter, but corn has so much natural sweetness and juiciness that you honestly don't need anything on it other than perhaps a splash of lemon juice. This makes a really healthy snack, but you can also slice off the corn kernels and scatter them on salads, soups, or stir-fries.

1 ear of corn
Lemon wedge for squeezing (optional)

Cut off the stalk end of the ear and peel away the husk and silk. Trim off the pointed end. Place a couple of paper towels on a large plate.

Bring a pan of water to a boil, then place the ear of corn in the pan and boil for about 5 minutes (until a kernel comes off the cob easily). Don't add salt to the pan—it is not only off the menu during the nine-day plan, but it will also toughen the corn.

Using tongs, transfer the corn to the paper towels to absorb any excess moisture. You can drizzle it with lemon juice if you like.

Main meals

These main meals have been split into cold meals and hot meals. The cold meals (starting on page 130) contain salads, sandwiches, dips, and even a raw soup, which make quick and easy lunches, and the hot meals (starting on page 136) include soups and stews, so that you can look forward to a warming, filling supper at the end of the day. These are flexible, however, so if the weather is warm and you feel like having salad for lunch and for supper, then do. Equally, if you want something hot at both meals, then have soup for lunch and stew for supper. The one rule we do insist on is that you have Super Greens Mix (opposite) with at least one main meal each day. This blend of parsley, basil, watercress, and baby spinach is a great way to eat far more greens and herbs than you normally would in a simple salad, and it will give your liver a huge boost. It also adds color and flavor to soups and stews.

Please note:

- this symbol indicates an oily fish recipe
- ✳ this symbol means the recipe is suitable for freezing

Detox Tip

Vegetarians and vegans who will not be eating the recommended three portions of oily fish in the nine-day plan should use omega-rich seed oils like hempseed or flaxseed oil to ensure that they obtain omega-3 fats.

Super Greens Mix SERVES 1

This blend of leafy greens and herbs is a brilliant way to dramatically increases your intake of these flavonoid- and vitamin C–rich ingredients without having to wade through buckets of salad. Simply blend it all together with some oil and lemon juice and serve it on soups, salads, and main meals. We recommend that you have a serving of this on at least one of your meals each day, and ideally two, to give your liver a helping hand. You can vary the greens and herbs used according to taste and availability. Add avocado (rich in vitamin E and protein) for a thicker consistency, or cucumber (a very cleansing vegetable) for a thinner texture. Equally, you can ring the changes by adding raw garlic (to get your daily intake of sulfurous vegetables), sun-dried tomatoes or roasted peppers, olives, marinated artichoke hearts, pumpkin seeds, or pine nuts.

1 large handful watercress
1 large handful baby spinach
1 large handful fresh basil leaves
1 large handful fresh flat-leaf parsley leaves
About 1 tablespoon extra-virgin olive oil or an omega-rich
    seed oil such as hempseed or flaxseed oil
Squeeze of fresh lemon juice, or to taste

Whiz all the ingredients together in a mini blender or food processor. If you don't have one of these handy, finely chop the herbs, then stir in the oil and lemon juice. The mixture should hold together a little like pesto.

Cold meals

These recipes can all be eaten cold, so they make ideal packed lunches to take to work or grab from the fridge. Some do involve a little cooking beforehand, but they are all simple and quick to prepare. You can choose from rye sandwiches, salads, and even a raw soup, which is perfect for summer.

Superboost Sesame Salad   SERVES 2

The strong flavors of toasted sesame oil and lemon juice breathe life into this easy-to-make salad without adding any salt or spices. Celery is rich in the mineral potassium, which helps to lower blood pressure, while the chickpeas provide phytoestrogens to help balance hormones, which in turn reduces strain on your liver to regulate levels. Double the quantities for a more substantial meal.

> 1 (14^1/$_2$-ounce) can chickpeas, drained and rinsed
> 2 celery stalks, finely chopped
> 6 marinated artichoke hearts, coarsely chopped
> 6 green onions, white and green parts, finely chopped
> 1 tablespoon raw sesame seeds
> 1 teaspoon toasted sesame oil, or to taste
> Juice of ^{1}/$_2$ lemon
> Mixed salad greens
> 2 servings Super Greens Mix (page 129; optional)

Mix all of the ingredients together and serve with the mixed salad greens, including a portion of Super Greens Mix, if you like, or if needed for your daily serving.

Superfood Sandwich for Beautiful Skin

SERVES 1

The salmon in this sandwich provides one of your recommended three servings of omega-3 essential fats during the nine-day plan. Both salmon and watercress are also excellent sources of zinc, which both men and women need for a healthy libido. What's more, watercress contains greater quantities of the antioxidant carotenoids lutein and zeaxanthin as well as vitamin C than apples and broccoli, to help mop up damaging free radicals. All in all, this truly is a superfood sandwich.

1 salmon fillet (preferably wild)
1/2 serving Super Greens Mix (page 129; also see Detox Tip)
1 large or 2 small slices pumpernickel-style rye bread
   (choose a yeast-free brand)
Squeeze of fresh lemon juice

Steam the salmon fillet for about 15 minutes until cooked (it should flake easily when pressed). Skin and flake (checking for bones as you do so) and allow it to cool.

Spread the greens mix on toasted rye bread (or untoasted if you prefer) and top with the flaked salmon and a squeeze of lemon juice.

Detox Tip

In your Super Greens Mix to accompany this recipe, do use watercress, as the peppery flavor is the perfect partner for salmon. Make sure you use enough oil to give this a pesto-type consistency for ease of spreading.

Skin-Defense Dip   SERVES 2

The eggplant and beans in this dip give a smoky, rich flavor to this delicious blend of vegetables. Cooked tomato products, such as tomato paste, are a better source of lycopene than raw tomatoes. This antioxidant nutrient not only helps to protect eyesight but also has been shown to reduce skin damage by ultraviolet rays by as much as 30 percent! Consider it an edible sunscreen to keep wrinkles at bay. Serve this dip with crudités and rice cakes or spread it on pumpernickel-style rye bread and top with watercress, arugula, or baby spinach.

1 teaspoon coconut oil or olive oil
1 clove garlic, crushed
1 red onion, diced
1/4 globe eggplant, cubed
1 tablespoon tomato paste
1 (14-ounce) can pinto or red beans, drained and rinsed
1 teaspoon low-sodium vegetable broth powder
2 servings Super Greens Mix (page 129)

Heat the oil in a skillet and sauté the garlic and onion for a couple of minutes to let the onion start to soften, then add the eggplant and cook for a few minutes until it browns and softens.

Add the tomato paste, beans, and broth powder and stir together.

Place the mixture in a food processor or blender and blend until fairly smooth. You can add the greens mix to the food processor with the other ingredients, or you can stir it in afterward.

Cleansing Bean and
Artichoke Salad

This dish is surprisingly filling and full flavored, and it is equally good served hot or cold. It is rich in the detox mineral sulfur, from the garlic and onions, as well as being packed with digestion-boosting fiber, including inulin in the artichokes, which encourages beneficial probiotic bacteria to flourish in the gut.

2 cloves garlic, crushed
1 red onion, finely diced
1 tablespoon coconut oil, or 2 tablespoons olive oil
1¹/₂ cups cherry tomatoes, chopped
2 tablespoons tomato paste
1 (14¹/₂-ounce) can mixed beans, drained and rinsed
6 marinated artichoke heart halves coarsely chopped
2 tablespoons black olives, pitted and coarsely chopped
   (optional)
1 handful fresh basil leaves, torn, or a dollop of
   Super Greens Mix (page 129)

Heat the oil in a skillet and sauté the garlic and onion for about 3 minutes until translucent.

Add the tomatoes and cook for a couple of minutes until they disintegrate.

Stir in the tomato paste, beans, artichoke hearts, and olives Lower the heat and simmer for about 5 minutes until thick and rich—you can add a splash of water to loosen it if the sauce dries up. Stir in the basil or greens mix just before serving.

Superfood Salad of Quinoa with
Roasted Vegetables   SERVES 2

Research has shown that consuming vitamin E and the nutrient lycopene together, as in the pumpkin seeds and tomatoes used here, enhances their positive antioxidant effects. Surprisingly, the antioxidant lycopene in tomatoes is more readily absorbed by the body when the tomatoes are cooked, so these roasted cherry tomatoes are ideal. Regular consumption of lycopene has been shown to reduce skin damage from ultraviolet rays from the sun. These benefits, combined with the zinc- and protein-rich quinoa and the liver-boosting herbs, makes for a superfood meal. Make this dish in advance and eat it cold or warm, but it is also delicious hot, either on its own or with arugula. Add some fresh lemon juice for a zesty flavor, if you like.

1 small unpeeled sweet potato, cubed
1 small red onion, coarsely chopped
1 red, yellow, or orange bell pepper, coarsely chopped
1 small zucchini, coarsely chopped
2 cloves garlic, thinly sliced
1 to 2 tablespoons olive oil
1 cup cherry tomatoes
1 cup quinoa
1 teaspoon low-sodium vegetable broth powder
2 cups boiling water
2 heaping tablespoons pumpkin seeds
2 servings Super Greens Mix (page 129)

Preheat the oven to 400°F. Place the sweet potato, onion, bell pepper, zucchini, and garlic in a roasting pan, drizzle with the oil, stir to coat, and roast for 40 minutes. Add the cherry tomatoes and return to the oven for 15 to 20 minutes until the tomato skins split and the sweet potatoes are soft when pierced.

Meanwhile, place the quinoa and broth powder in a saucepan and add the boiling water. Bring to a boil, then cover, reduce the heat, and simmer for 12 to 15 minutes until the liquid is absorbed and the grains are fluffy. Set aside, covered, while the vegetables finish cooking.

Five minutes before the vegetables are done, spread the pumpkin seeds in a pie tin and pop them in the oven on the top shelf to toast.

Stir the roasted vegetables and the greens mix into the quinoa, then sprinkle the toasted pumpkin seeds on top. Let cool, or eat warm, if you prefer.

Raw Summer Soup   SERVES 2

This soup maximizes the nutrient content of its ingredients, as they are served raw. Cucumber and lemons are both very cleansing for the liver, whereas the avocado and olive oil provide heart-friendly monounsaturated fat. Avocados are also rich in vitamin E, which helps to keep your skin in good condition.

1 avocado, pitted and flesh scooped from the skin
$1/2$ cucumber, coarsely chopped
1 cup cherry tomatoes
1 small handful fresh basil leaves
2 tablespoons cold-pressed oil (extra-virgin olive oil
    or flaxseed or hempseed oil)
Juice of $1/4$ lemon
2 green onions, white and green parts, finely sliced on the
    diagonal, or 2 servings Super Greens Mix (page 129)

Using a blender, puree the avocado, cucumber, tomatoes, basil, and oil together until smooth, then pour into bowls and sprinkle with the green onions or spoon on the greens mix. Eat immediately or chill until ready to serve.

Hot meals

Here are some warming, filling recipes for comfort food during your detox. There is no need to go hungry when you are avoiding foods like meat, dairy products, and wheat—we have included masses of fresh, wholesome ingredients to help nourish you back to health. These are intended as suppers, when you have a little more time, but the stews and soups could also be eaten for lunch.

Patrick's Primordial Soup   SERVES 2 TO 3

This soup was designed by Patrick to help his wife, Gaby, get over a virus, and it's now highly regarded as a renowned health tonic by his readers! It is called primordial because it contains foods that provide the key nutrients to ensure good health. It is incredibly rich in vitamin E and beta-carotene, as well as anti-inflammatory onions, garlic, and ginger. The coconut milk not only gives a rich, creamy flavor, it also contains medium-chain triglycerides: a special kind of saturated fat that isn't stored as fat but is used to give you energy. Coconut is also thought to help thyroid function and to fight infection.

1 tablespoon coconut oil or olive oil
1/2 red onion, coarsely chopped
1 clove garlic, crushed
1 large or 2 small to medium carrots, peeled and chopped
1 large or 2 small to medium unpeeled sweet potatoes, chopped to the same size as the carrot
1 heaping teaspoon grated fresh ginger
1/4 teaspoon ground turmeric
2 teaspoons reduced-sodium vegetable broth powder
1/2 red bell pepper, diced
5 tablespoons coconut milk (shake the can before opening, as it separates)
2 to 3 servings Super Greens Mix (page 129)

Heat the oil in a large skillet and gently sauté the onion and garlic for a few minutes until they start to soften but do not turn brown.

Add the carrots, sweet potatoes, ginger, turmeric, and broth powder. Add boiling water to cover and bring to a boil. Cover and simmer for about 15 minutes until the vegetables are soft.

Add the bell pepper and coconut milk. Transfer to a blender in batches and puree until smooth and thick. Stir 1 serving of greens mix into each serving of soup.

Baked Sweet Potatoes with Bean Stew
SERVES 2

Sweet potatoes are incredibly rich in the antioxidant vitamins beta-carotene and vitamin E, both of which are required to keep the immune system functioning and to keep skin in good condition. They are deliciously smooth and sweet when baked, and make a very filling, warming meal when topped with this rich, thick ragout-style bean stew.

2 large sweet potatoes
Olive oil for coating

STEW
1 tablespoon coconut oil or olive oil
2 cloves garlic, crushed
1 large red onion, diced
4 ounces cremini mushrooms, sliced (see Cook's Tip, on page 138)
2 tablespoons tomato paste
1 (14-ounce) can plum tomatoes
1 (14-ounce) can pinto or red beans, drained and rinsed
1/2 teaspoon reduced-sodium vegetable broth powder
1/2 teaspoon herbes de Provence, or to taste
Freshly ground pepper

Preheat the oven to 400°F. Prick the potatoes all over. Rub with a little oil and place on a baking sheet. Bake for 1 hour until soft all the way through when pierced with a knife. Meanwhile, prepare the stew. Heat the oil in a skillet and gently sauté the garlic and onion for 2 minutes, then add the mushrooms and cook for 5 minutes until fairly soft.

Add the remaining ingredients and simmer for 5 to 10 minutes to allow the vegetables to soften and the sauce to thicken. Check the seasoning and adjust if necessary.

Open up the baked potatoes and spoon the stew inside.

Cook's Tip

To clean mushrooms, wipe them with a soft brush or a piece of paper towel.

Leek, Cannellini, and Potato Soup

SERVES 2

This is a slight twist on a classic that will fill you up and boost flagging energy levels. Leeks are a good source of prebiotics, which provide fuel for the digestion and immune system to boost probiotic bacteria. They also, along with the garlic, provide sulfur to assist your liver's detox capacity. We have added high-fiber, low-glycemic-load cannellini beans to help thicken the soup and create a creamy consistency.

1 teaspoon coconut oil or olive oil
2 cloves garlic, crushed
2 large leeks, white parts only, sliced and well rinsed
2 medium or 3 small unpeeled new potatoes, cubed
2 cups boiling water
1 tablespoon reduced-sodium vegetable broth powder
1 (14-ounce) can cannellini or Great Northern beans, drained and
   rinsed
Freshly ground pepper
2 servings Super Greens Mix (page 129) if required for daily serving

Heat the oil in a skillet and sauté the garlic for 30 seconds. Add the leeks, cover, and cook for 3 minutes until they start to soften.

Stir in the potatoes, water, and broth powder. Cover and simmer for 15 minutes.

Add the beans and blend with a handheld blender, or transfer to a blender in batches and puree until fairly smooth. Season with pepper, then add a dollop of greens mix.

Cook's Tip

Beans are a better source of carbohydrate than potatoes for anyone with blood sugar imbalances, such as diabetics or sugar addicts. As they are digested slowly, they cause a gradual rise in blood sugar in contrast to the rapid but short-lived burst of energy from potatoes. Beans are also recommended for clearing arteries, in part because of their choline content, which is used for fat metabolism. Their high fiber content makes beans excellent for preventing constipation.

Age-Defying Carrot and
Lentil Soup

SERVES 4

Thick and filling, this soup is perfect to keep in the fridge ready for an instant meal. The bright orange color shows how rich this soup is in the antioxidant vitamin beta-carotene, which will mop up free radicals to prevent them from damaging cells. Lentils provide more folic acid than any other unfortified food. Folic acid is not only important for pregnant women, it is also a vital nutrient for everyone, as it helps reduce your risk of age-related degenerative diseases.

    1 tablespoon coconut oil or olive oil
    2 cloves garlic, crushed
    1 onion, coarsely chopped
    2 large celery stalks, sliced
    4 medium to large carrots, peeled and sliced
    1 cup red lentils, rinsed
    4 cups hot vegetable broth (see Cook's Tip)

Heat the oil in a large skillet and sauté the garlic and onion for 5 minutes to soften.

Add the celery, carrots, lentils, and broth, then stir and bring to a boil. Cover and simmer for 10 minutes to allow the carrots to soften. Using a handheld blender, or blending in batches in a regular blender, puree until smooth or to your preferred consistency.

Cook's Tip

For a quick stock, combine 4 cups boiling water with 1 tablespoon reduced-sodium vegetable broth powder. Freeze or chill any leftovers.

Mushroom and Pine Nut–Stuffed Peppers

Peppers are very high in antioxidants and vitamin C, and delicious as served here. To make this even healthier, choose shiitake mushrooms for their lentinan content, as this polysaccharide is a powerful immune booster long used in traditional Chinese medicine.

2 large red bell peppers
1 tablespoon coconut oil or olive oil
1 yellow onion, finely chopped
2 cloves garlic, crushed
5 ounces cremini or stemmed shiitake mushrooms, sliced
1 teaspoon reduced-sodium vegetable broth powder
1 cup cooked brown basmati rice
1 tablespoon pine nuts (see Cook's Tip)
1 handful fresh basil leaves, chopped

Preheat the oven to 400°F. Cut the tops off the peppers (reserving them to make lids) and remove the seeds and veins.

Heat the oil in a skillet and gently sauté the onion and garlic for 2 minutes. Add the mushrooms and broth powder and sauté for 2 to 3 minutes.

Transfer to a large bowl and add the rice, nuts, and basil.

Stuff the peppers with the mixture and place the tops back on.

Place on a baking sheet and bake for 35 minutes, or until tender and heated through.

Cook's Tip

Pine nuts taste wonderful in this dish, but are expensive. Cheaper alternatives include chopped walnuts or cashews, or sliced almonds. Or use sunflower or pumpkin seeds for a nut-free version.

Rice with Super Greens Pesto   SERVES 2

A cross between a pesto and a tapenade, the combination of olives and herbs in the sauce for this dish adds flavor and texture as well as replenishing your nutrient levels, of course. The pumpkin seeds provide protein and zinc, while the olives are not only a good source of heart-friendly monounsaturated fats but are also rich in vitamin E as well as flavonoids, both of which appear to have anti-inflammatory properties. Serve with a large green salad that includes some tomato and thinly sliced red onion for color. If you have more time, sautéed or broiled zucchini makes an attractive and delicious accompaniment. Thinly slice them lengthwise and marinate for 10 minutes in a little lemon juice and olive oil before lightly sautéing or broiling for 30 seconds or so.

3/4 cup brown basmati rice, rinsed
1 1/2 cups water

SUPER GREENS PESTO
    2 servings Super Greens Mix (page 129)
    2 tablespoons pumpkin seeds, toasted for about
        2 minutes in a dry skillet
    6 tablespoons kalamata olives, pitted
    2 tablespoons extra-virgin olive oil (from the olive jar
        if the olives are packed in oil)
    2 large cloves garlic, crushed
    4 handfuls fresh basil leaves
    2 handfuls arugula
    2 handfuls baby spinach or fresh flat-leaf parsley leaves
    Freshly ground pepper
    Juice of 1 lemon, or to taste

In a small saucepan, bring the water to a boil and stir in the rice. Reduce the heat to a simmer, cover, and cook until al dente, 20 to 30 minutes.

Meanwhile, prepare the pesto: Blend all the ingredients together in a blender or food processor. Taste to check the flavor—you can add more of any of the ingredients to tweak the flavor, if you like. Stir the pesto into the rice. Serve warm.

Fennel and Mixed Rice Pilaf   SERVES 2

This dish has a subtle mixture of flavors and textures, from the soft, slightly sweet fennel and onion to the crunchy wild rice. Fennel is an excellent liver booster, and wild rice provides more protein and minerals than standard rice. The recipe is delicious cold; you can eat this for supper and then take some to work the next day for lunch.

    1 teaspoon reduced-sodium vegetable broth powder
    $^1/_2$ cup mixed rice (wild rice, brown basmati rice, and
        red rice; see Cook's Tip)
    1 tablespoon coconut oil or olive oil
    1 small or $^1/_2$ large red onion, cut into thin wedges
    $^1/_2$ fennel bulb, trimmed and thinly sliced lengthwise
    5 ounces cremini mushrooms, quartered
    1 (14-ounce) can green lentils, drained and rinsed
    1 tablespoon freshly squeezed lemon juice
    2 tablespoons minced fresh flat-leaf parsley
    Freshly ground pepper

Bring a large saucepan of water to a boil and add the broth powder. Add the rice, reduce the heat to a simmer, cover, and cook for 20 to 30 minutes until al dente. As the grains are unrefined, they should be tender when cooked but will still retain some bite. Drain the rice.

While the rice is cooking, heat the oil in a medium skillet over medium-high heat and sauté the onion, fennel, and mushrooms for 5 to 10 minutes until they soften. Turn off the heat.

Add the rice to the pan of vegetables along with the lentils and stir over medium-low heat. Stir in the lemon juice, parsley, and lots of pepper. Taste to check the seasoning before serving.

Cook's Tip

You can buy mixed rice in natural foods stores, or you could make up your own combination.

Trout en Papillote with Roasted Vegetables

SERVES 2

Cooking fish en papillote (in a parchment paper packet) preserves all of its juices, flavor, and essential fats. This recipe is bursting with color, from the orange-fleshed sweet potatoes to the vibrant green of the greens mix, all of which contribute to its high anti-oxidant content. The garlic, parsley, and lemon juice all provide flavor as well as nutrients: garlic is rich in sulfur and is a powerful anti-inflammatory, while parsley and lemons are rich in vitamin C.

2 medium or 1 large unpeeled sweet potato,
    cut into fairly thin wedges
2 zucchini, cut into similar-sized wedges
About 1 tablespoon olive oil
2 rainbow trout (preferably organic), filleted
2 cloves garlic, crushed
Juice of 1 lemon
2 teaspoons minced fresh flat-leaf parsley
2 servings Super Greens Mix (page 129)

Preheat the oven to 350°F. Place the sweet potato and zucchini in a roasting pan, drizzle with the oil, and roast for about 1 hour, turning the vegetables over halfway through, until the sweet potato is soft when pierced with a knife.

Meanwhile, cut a piece of parchment paper large enough to cover both fish lying diagonally across the center of the paper when it is folded in half on the diagonal.

Season the inside of each fish with the garlic, lemon juice, and parsley and place the fish diagonally across the center of the parchment paper. Fold the paper in half to make a triangle.

Starting from one end, gradually fold up the edges to seal the paper into a packet, overlapping each fold slightly over the last fold to keep it from unraveling.

Place the packet on a baking sheet and bake for 25 minutes. Unwrap carefully to avoid being burned by the steam, then divide the fish and cooked vegetables between two plates and add a portion of greens mix to each. Serve immediately.

Cook's Tip

The reason we suggest you bake the fish in parchment paper rather than aluminum foil is that the aluminum in foil can leach into your food, particularly if it comes into contact with acidic ingredients such as the lemon juice in this recipe. Some evidence points to high aluminum levels being implicated in Alzheimer's disease.

Salmon with French
Green Lentils

Here is another omega-3-rich fish dish to keep your essential-fat levels up during the detox plan, as well as providing protein to fuel your liver's detoxification pathways and your body's repair work. Steaming the salmon helps to preserve as much of the valuable omega-3 fats as possible, because it is a much gentler cooking technique than the direct, fierce heat from a skillet or grill. French green lentils not only hold their shape when cooked, providing texture to the dish, but they are also very rich in protein, and are combined here with antioxidant-dense tomato paste and sulfur-rich leeks to create a filling and nutritious stew to serve with the salmon. The dish is also delicious cold.

2/3 cup green lentils, well rinsed
1 1/3 cups water
2 teaspoons reduced-sodium vegetable broth powder
2 leeks, white part only, finely sliced and well rinsed
2 salmon fillets (preferably wild), pin bones removed
2 tablespoons tomato paste
Squeeze of fresh lemon juice
2 servings Super Greens Mix (page 129)
Freshly ground pepper

Place the lentils in a medium saucepan and add the water and broth powder. Bring to a boil, then lower the heat to a simmer, cover, and cook for 20 to 25 minutes until the lentils are al dente, adding the leeks to the pan halfway through cooking. The lentils will absorb most of the liquid during cooking.

Put the salmon in a steamer, cover, and cook over boiling water for about 15 minutes or until the flesh flakes easily when pressed. (Alternatively, if you don't have steamer, put the fish in a skillet, cover with water, and simmer gently until the flesh flakes when pressed.)

Stir the tomato paste into the lentil mixture, along with a splash of water and squeeze of lemon juice to loosen the consistency and produce a thick stew.

Either serve the salmon on a bed of stew and spoon the greens mix over the top, or fold the greens mix into the stew before topping with the fish. Sprinkle with pepper.

Desserts

These desserts serve two purposes: first, to increase your fruit and antioxidant intake, and second, to keep your morale high during the nine-day detox plan when you are cutting out other foods. We recommend that you have a dessert on each of the weekends—one at the start of the detox and the other at the end—to spread out your treats and give you something to look forward to, but it is entirely up to you when you include them. The recipes have not only passed testers' stringent taste tests, but they are also a valuable source of vitamins, fiber, and other plant nutrients, plus protein to enable your liver to detoxify efficiently.

Detox Pear and
Blueberry Crumble

Here's a comfort-food dessert to cheer you up if you are going through sugar withdrawal symptoms. Standard crumbles are high in refined wheat, butter, and sugar, but our liver-friendly version replaces flour with oats and almonds and is dairy free and sugar free. It is rich in vitamins, minerals, and fiber to help digestion and detoxification. Ginger not only adds a warming flavor, it is also a very effective natural anti-inflammatory, while cinnamon helps improve glucose tolerance to balance blood sugar levels.

2 medium to large unpeeled pears, cored and coarsely chopped
1 cup fresh or frozen blueberries
Ground ginger and/or ground cinnamon

TOPPING
2 tablespoons coconut oil or olive oil
1 tablespoon xylitol (a naturally occurring sugar alternative
    that does not upset blood sugar levels)
^{2}/$_3$ cup old-fashioned rolled oats
2 heaping tablespoons ground almonds (almond meal)
2 tablespoons sliced almonds or coarsely chopped nuts
    such as pecans, hazelnuts, or walnuts, or pumpkin seeds
    or sunflower seeds

Place the fruit in a saucepan with a splash of water, cover, and cook gently for about 5 minutes until the fruit softens, stirring from time to time. You can add more water if the fruit starts to stick to the bottom of the pan. Add ginger and/or cinnamon to taste.

Meanwhile, make the topping by gently heating the oil and xylitol in a small skillet. Stir in the oats and toast gently for a few minutes until they start to crisp.

Mix in the ground and sliced almonds (or other nuts or seeds) and remove from the heat.

Spoon the stewed fruit into bowls and sprinkle with the topping.

Fruit Burst Frozen Yogurt   SERVES 4

This dessert does contain dairy products, which are otherwise to be avoided on the nine-day detox, but the organic, live-culture natural yogurt provides valuable probiotic bacteria, which will give your digestive and immune systems a boost. Probiotics populate the gut wall to prevent harmful bacteria from taking hold. The creamy yogurt also helps to give the same smooth texture as a sorbet or ice cream. The berries are packed with vitamin C and bioflavonoids, all of which will replenish your body's own levels.

14 ounces frozen mixed berries
1³/4 cups live-culture natural yogurt
¹/4 cup xylitol (see page 148), or to taste

In a blender, combine all the ingredients and puree until smooth and the consistency of sorbet or frozen yogurt. Eat quickly before it melts (although if it does melt, it makes a delicious drink).

Cook's Tip

Let the frozen berries defrost for a few minutes first if your blender won't cope with fully frozen ones.

Juices and smoothies

If your only experience of juices and smoothies is via the concentrated orange juice found in supermarket cartons or the pasteurized smoothies sold in bottles, you are missing out. Fresh fruit juice has a vitalizing quality and a fantastic taste, just as a smoothie straight from the blender has an invigorating freshness that is so much nicer than even premium brands of smoothies made using pasteurized fruit. It goes without saying that these increasingly fashionable health drinks are also incredibly good sources of vitamins, minerals, and phytonutrients—that is, nutrients derived from plants. What is more, they are very easy to digest and absorb, so they are ideal for anyone whose liver is struggling to cope with a toxic overload, or who is ill or recovering from an illness or injury. For these reasons, we recommend you have a fresh juice or smoothie each day of the nine-day plan (and beyond if you wish) to give your body a regular nutrient burst. Just one word of warning: Some fruits are higher in fruit sugars than others, chiefly tropical fruits like mangos, lychees, pineapple, bananas, passion fruit, and Hachiya persimmons. Juicing extracts the sugars and leaves the fiber, so the sugar is even more rapidly absorbed than by eating the whole fruit. While this is not a problem during the nine-day detox plan, where the focus is on replenishing nutrients and maintaining energy while you omit many other foods, over the long term it is advisable to limit the amount of high-sugar fruits you eat in favor of lower-sugar ones, which release their sugar more slowly to keep blood sugar balanced.

Equipment
The following items will enable you to make all manner of drinks using every kind of fruit or vegetable imaginable:

* Juice extractor (juicer)
* Citrus press, for citrus fruits like oranges, lemons, grapefruits, and limes (optional)
* Handheld or regular blender

Juicers vary in price from the very reasonable to much more sophisticated models with price tags to match. If you find you are getting in the habit of juicing daily, it is worth investing in a good model, as they have stronger motors to withstand regular, heavy use, and extract more juice, and therefore more nutrients, from the fruit.

If you are on a budget, the one item that is essential out of these three is the blender, as not only can you use this to make smoothies, but it is also incredibly useful for pureeing soups and the Super Greens Mix that we recommend you add to main meals (page 129).

Ingredients

The only limit to flavors and combinations of smoothies and juices is your imagination. The possibilities are endless, from a freshly squeezed orange juice to a cooling Caribbean cocktail of coconut milk, banana, and mango with crushed ice. The one point that we cannot stress strongly enough, however, is the quality of your ingredients. Where possible, choose organic fruits and vegetables in order to limit your intake of toxic pesticides and waxes that are routinely used on commercial produce. Organic food is also richer in vitamins and minerals than intensively produced fruits and vegetables that have been grown in nutrient-depleted soil and artificially ripened before being stored for long periods. That said, organic apples grown in New Zealand will not contain as much goodness as those that are grown locally, even if they are not, strictly speaking, organic. The best way to shop is to choose fruits and vegetables that have been grown nearby when they are in season, to cut down on travel time. Supermarkets are increasingly stocking local produce, but other places to look include produce markets, farmers' markets, and local grocery stores, or you may wish to invest in a weekly organic delivery box from a community supported agriculture (CSA) farm to keep you well stocked with fresh ingredients.

You should also thoroughly wash all ingredients that do not need peeling. If you are not using organic fruits and vegetables, try rinsing produce with a "veggie wash" (available from natural foods stores) to remove much of the pesticides and sprays.

Storage

The whole point of a juice or smoothie is to give your body a short, sharp burst of nutrients. These nutrients are delicate, however, and are depleted by time spent exposed to light, air, and heat. Therefore, the sooner you drink your juice or smoothie after processing, the better. If you need to prepare a drink in advance to take to work, then do it that morning rather than the day before, and store it in the fridge or in a chilled container. Add a squeeze of lemon juice to the mixture to prevent it from oxidizing and turning brown.

Fruit

Think beyond the usual choices and add some different colors and flavors to your drinks by using a variety of different ingredients. The more vivid the color, the higher the nutrient content, so apply the Rainbow Rule to your shopping: Choose as many different colors of fruits and vegetables as possible, as each color indicates a different kind of plant nutrient. Some ideas for your shopping basket include:

Apples

Apricots

Bananas

Berries (including strawberries, raspberries, blueberries, blackberries, currants, cranberries)

Cherries

Grapefruit, especially pink

Grapes

Guavas

Kiwifruit

Lemons

Limes

Mangos

Melons (all types, including watermelon, honeydew, cantaloupe)

Nectarines

Oranges

Papayas

Passion fruit

Peaches

Pears

Pineapples

Plums

Pomegranates

Tangerines, clementines, satsumas

Tomatoes

Limit high-sugar fruits:

Bananas (eat no more frequently than 1 every other day)

Figs

Grapes

Guavas

Hachiya persimmons

Kiwifruits

Lychees

Mangos

Passion fruit

Pineapples

Vegetables

Juice from the following vegetables and herbs can be drunk raw, straight from the juicer, even ones like parsnips, which you may be more used to seeing served up at Sunday lunch:

Arugula	Cucumbers
Baby spinach	Ginger
Basil	Kale
Beets	Lettuce
Broccoli (or, preferably, broccolini)	Mint
	Parsley
Cabbage	Parsnips
Carrots	Peppers
Cauliflower	Sweet potatoes
Celery	Watercress

Juices

Here are some classic but delicious juice combinations to get you started and to inspire you to create your own favorites.

Invigorator SERVES 1

Not only do the berries sweeten the otherwise tart grapefruit, but their vibrant color also provides plant-based nutrients like flavonoids, which help to fight infection. Phytonutrients in grapefruit called limonoids also promote the formation of the detoxifying enzyme glutathione S-transferase, to help inhibit tumors.

1 pink grapefruit
1 handful fresh or frozen berries (such as
   blueberries, raspberries, or strawberries)

Push each ingredient through a juicer according to the manufacturer's instructions.

Skin Nourisher SERVES 1

Simple and sweet, this mixture is extremely good for the complexion thanks to the vitamin C in the apple, from which the body makes collagen, and the beta-carotene in the carrot, which helps disarm free radicals to prevent wrinkles and sun damage. You could also use this as a base to which you could add other ingredients, such as lemon juice and ginger, or celery and cucumber.

1 large apple
1 carrot

Push each ingredient through a juicer according to the manufacturer's instructions.

C-Sharp
SERVES 1

This juice is an immune booster that is packed with vitamin C from both the apple and lemon, and the celery is rich in potassium, which helps to lower blood pressure. If you are not a fan of celery don't worry—its flavor is overpowered by the sweet apple and sharp lemon juice.

1 celery stalk
1 large apple
$^1/_2$ lemon (or add the juice separately for a sweeter version)

Push each ingredient through a juicer according to the manufacturer's instructions.

Stomach Settler
SERVES 1

All the ingredients in this juice can soothe and heal a troubled digestive tract. Pineapple contains the digestive enzyme bromelain, which helps you break down your food and also has strong anti-inflammatory properties. The lemon and ginger add a refreshingly zingy flavor.

1 carrot
1 pear
2 thick slices fresh pineapple (about $^1/_4$ of a medium fruit)
$^1/_2$ lemon (or add the juice separately for a sweeter version)
$^1/_4$ teaspoon grated fresh ginger

Push the carrot, pear, pineapple, and lemon through a juicer according to the manufacturer's instructions. Stir in the ginger.

Smoothies

Preparing a smoothie is even easier making than a juice, as you simply blend and serve. You can use banana to thicken drinks, but remember that you should not have a banana more than once every other day, as they are high in starch, which will raise your blood sugar rapidly. Other ways to add a creamy consistency include coconut milk or nondairy milks such as unsweetened rice, soy, quinoa, almond, and oat milks. Here are a couple of suggestions to get you started.

Summer Fizz   SERVES 1

Strawberries and lemons are incredibly rich in vitamin C, and the sweet-sharp flavor combination makes this drink very refreshing. Make this smoothie in the summer months, however, when strawberries are in season; otherwise you will be paying a premium for flavorless imported varieties that are of negligible nutritional value (or use frozen berries). We also recommend naturally sparkling mineral water, as artificially carbonated ones are very abrasive to tooth enamel.

About 1 cup fresh or frozen strawberries
1 tablespoon freshly squeezed lemon juice
2 teaspoons xylitol (see page 148), or to taste
$^1/_2$ cup naturally sparkling (not carbonated) mineral water

Using a blender, puree the strawberries and lemon juice until smooth. Stir in the xylitol until it has dissolved, then stir in the mineral water.

Berry Tasty

This dairy-free smoothie gets its rich, creamy texture from the tahini, which also provides protein to keep your liver detoxing efficiently. Vary the flavor by using strawberries or blueberries instead of raspberries, or a mixture of all three. Xylitol, a safe sugar substitute sourced from plants, not only does not disrupt blood sugar levels but is also naturally antibacterial to help prevent tooth decay.

$1/2$ cup fresh or frozen raspberries
1 tablespoon tahini (sesame paste)
1 tablespoon xylitol
$1/2$ cup water

Using a blender, puree all the ingredients together.

Watermelon Whiz

Its high water content makes watermelon very refreshing and hydrating, while the deep color indicates that is is rich in nutrients, including beta-carotene for eye and skin health. The seeds should be kept in as they blend invisibly into the drink yet provide a powerful vitamin E and enzyme punch.

1 medium slice watermelon, trimmed of rind, about 8 ounces

Using a blender, puree the watermelon, seeds and all, until smooth. Serve with ice or blend crushed ice with the watermelon for an instant chilled juice.

Cool Caribbean   SERVES 1

Bananas are full of the mineral potassium, which helps lower blood pressure. They are also full of fiber for aiding digestion, and the fat from the coconut is used as energy rather than being stored as fat. Remember that you should not have more than one banana every other day on the 9-Day Liver Detox, however.

1 banana
1 large handful fresh or frozen strawberries
3/4 cup coconut milk (shake the can before opening, as it separates)
3 ice cubes

Using a blender, puree all the ingredients together and drink immediately.

Chapter Seven

Your Liver Detox for Life

Well done! You've completed your 9-Day Liver Detox, and I hope you are feeling much better. Many people experience such a shift in health, energy, mood, and mental clarity that they wonder, "Should I be eating like this all the time?" Of course, the answer is yes, but being this strict with your diet all the time is neither easy nor necessary.

The first few days post-detox can be difficult. Don't imagine that you can just go back to your old way of eating and drinking immediately, because your body will rebel. Introduce excluded foods one at a time and slowly, eating no more than the quantities I recommend and chewing well, but don't give up any of the foods you have been eating on the detox diet. Reintroduce the foods in the order I suggest below, and if there are any bad reactions, just remove the food you introduced last and move on to the next one. This is the time when you can test whether you are indeed sensitive to any of the excluded foods and identify which ones they are. Here's how you do it.

Reintroducing milk

The first food to reintroduce is milk. Have the equivalent of a large glass of it, or cheese or yogurt, or all of them, on the first day after the nine days' detox. Apart from that, stick to your detox diet. Notice how you feel over the next forty-eight hours. Particularly notice any digestive symptoms, breathing difficulties, stuffed-up nose, headaches, skin itching, or joint aches. If you do get such symptoms, there's a good chance you are allergic to milk. Ideally, get yourself tested (see Resources), but certainly keep avoiding milk products.

Few dairy-allergic people react to butter, since it's almost all fat and it's the protein in milk that people react to. Also, most dairy-allergic people also react to goat's and sheep's milk products.

In any event, I don't recommend anyone having dairy products every day. Ideally, keep your milk intake down to 2 cups a week and eat plenty of seeds, nuts, beans, and lentils as sources of calcium.

Reintroducing wheat

Wheat is the second food to reintroduce, and with it often comes yeast. On the third day after the detox, have your first slice of bread—in fact, why not have three?—one or two for breakfast and a nice sandwich for lunch. Notice how you feel over the next forty-eight hours. Particularly notice any digestive symptoms, bloating, stuffed-up nose, headaches, brain fog, mood dips, skin itching, or joint aches. If you do get such symptoms, there's a good chance you are allergic to either wheat or yeast. Ideally, get yourself tested (see Resources), but certainly keep avoiding wheat products and yeast for now. By the way, if you seem to be fine on pasta but worse on bread, that's an indication that you are sensitive to yeast.

If you don't react, then my advice is not to have wheat or other gluten grains every day, but often choose nongluten grains instead (see page 37). If you rotate a food, eating it no more than every four days, you are much less likely to become allergic to it.

Reintroducing alcohol

You might have been inclined to break open the champagne on completing your 9-Day Liver Detox—and why not? You deserve it. However, the reason I recommend reintroducing wheat and milk first is that alcohol increases your allergic potential by irritating the gut. So I wanted you to have the opportunity to test your sensitivity to wheat and milk before alcohol.

If you want to reintroduce alcohol and measure its effects on you, it is best to choose a yeast-free drink, such as champagne or spirits (a margarita with fresh lime juice is probably the best choice). Have a glass or two for three days in a row and notice how it makes you feel. Notice how you feel in the morning, your energy, mental clarity, motivation, mood, and digestion. Also, notice your cravings. Personally, I would recommend drinking no more than three times a week—ideally no more than one glass or unit—for optimum health. You may find that you feel worse after beer or wine, both of which contain yeast. If so, the chances are you're yeast sensitive.

Reintroducing meat

It's quite rare to be allergic to meat but it can happen. Meat is tough on the digestive system, particularly after a two-week break, so eat only a small amount at the first meal. Start with chicken and build up to red meats slowly. Meat will alter the acid–alkaline balance in your body for the worse, so don't decrease the fruits and vegetables, as they will counter the effect of the meat.

Reintroducing caffeine

Many people experience so much more energy after a detox that they simply don't need the short-term energy boost that caffeine gives, and therefore don't crave it. If so, the best course of action is to stay caffeine free. If, on the other hand, you want to test its effects, have a strong cup of coffee and notice how it makes you feel. Notice your mood, aggression, mental clarity, and cravings the next day. Caffeine is very addictive, and once you start having it every day you'll crave it every day. However, having the odd cup of tea or infrequent coffee is not a big deal, as long as it doesn't become habit-forming. Certainly don't exceed one coffee a day, two cups of tea, or three green teas on a regular basis. It's good to give caffeine a total break every now and then just to make sure you're not getting dependent on it.

Reintroducing bad fats and fried foods

. . . but it's better if you don't. Generally, it's best to stay away from fried foods and processed fat, as they damage your cell membranes, preventing nutrients from getting in and waste products from being removed. However, they are not addictive, nor do they cause allergic reactions. So, my advice is generally to avoid deep-fried foods and junk food high in processed or hydrogenated fats. However, the odd indulgence is not going to kill you.

How to use your liver detox for life

If you've achieved what you set out to achieve and your detox score (see page 83) has dropped substantially, then the question is how to make the habits you have learned into your habits for life.

My advice is to follow the 80/20 rule. That is, stick to the detox diet principles 80 percent of the time and be less strict with yourself 20 percent of the time. In practical terms, what this means is:

- Drink at least $4^1/2$ cups, or six 6-ounce glasses, of water every day

- Have a superfood twice a day

- Have three servings of antioxidant-rich foods a day, including cruciferous vegetables

- Eat wheat and milk products no more than once every four days

* Have alcohol or caffeinated drinks every five days (that means six times a month)
* Have seeds six days out of seven
* Take supplements every day

Supplements for super health

Once you've completed your 9-Day Liver Detox, which you may wish to extend to thirty days, there is no need to keep taking the additional supplements, but every reason to continue with the basics:

* A high-potency multivitamin and multimineral
* 1 to 2 grams of vitamin C, plus bioflavonoids found in berry extracts
* Essential omega-3 (EPA and DHA) and omega-6 (GLA) fats

Good multivitamins state on the pack "take twice a day," not only because you can't get enough in a single tablet unless you make it a horse pill but also because taking supplements twice a day is more effective. This is because the water-soluble vitamins B and C are only available in the body for up to six hours. So, your basic daily supplement program should look like the following. Remember to take supplements every day at breakfast and lunchtime.

	DOSAGE	
	Breakfast	Lunch
High-potency multivitamin	1	1
Vitamin C	1	1
Essential fats (EPA, DHA, and GLA)	1	

We hope that your experiences during the 9-Day Liver Detox have both helped you regain health and also helped you to learn what kind of diet and lifestyle suit you best, and that it has given you the tools and the inspiration to stick to it. If you ever do feel like you are going downhill, make a resolution to do another 9-Day Liver Detox and get your health back on track!

Notes

Chapter 1

1. Kaya, H., et al. 2008. The protective effect of N-acetylcysteine against cyclosporine A-induced hepatotoxicity in rats. *Journal of Applied Toxicology* 28(1): 15–20. Ruffmann, R., and A. Wendel. 1991. GSH rescue by N-acetylcysteine. *Klinische Wochenschrift* 69: 857–62. Woo, O., et al. 2000. Shorter duration of oral N-acetylcysteine therapy for acute acetaminophen overdose. *Annals of Emergency Medicine* 35(4): 363–68. Flora, S. 1999. Arsenic-induced oxidative stress and its reversibility following combined administration of N-acetylcysteine and meso 2,3-dimercaptosuccinic acid in rats. *Clinical and Experimental Pharmacology and Physiology* 26(11): 865–69. Makin, A., et al. 1995. 7-year experience of severe acetaminophen-induced hepatotoxicity (1987–1993). *Gastroenterology* 109(6): 1907–16. Villa, P., and P. Ghezzi. 1995. Effect of N-acetylcysteine on sepsis in mice *European Journal of Pharmacology* 292(3–4): 341–44.

2. Weber, C., et al. 1994. Effect of dietary coenzyme Q10 as an antioxidant in human plasma. *Molecular Aspects of Medicine* 15(Suppl): S97–102.

3. Schils, M., and J. Olson. 1994. *Modern Nutrition in Health & Disease*, 8th ed. Lea & Febiger. 432–48. Schwedhelm, E.,

et al. 2003. Clinical pharmacokinetics of antioxidants and their impact on systemic oxidative stress. *Clinical Pharmacokinetics* 42(5): 437–59.

4. Schils, M., and J. Olson. 1994. *Modern Nutrition in Health & Disease*, 8th ed. Lea & Febiger. 432–48. Schwedhelm, E., et al. 2003. Clinical pharmacokinetics of antioxidants and their impact on systemic oxidative stress. *Clinical Pharmacokinetics* 42(5): 437–59. Van Haaften, R. I., et al. 2003. Effect of vitamin E on glutathione-dependent enzymes. *Drug Metabolism Reviews* 35(2–3): 215–53.

5. Schwedhelm, E., et al. 2003. Clinical pharmacokinetics of antioxidants and their impact on systemic oxidative stress. *Clinical Pharmacokinetics* 42(5): 437–59.

6. Ibid.

7. Touvier, M., et al. 2005. Dual association of beta-carotene with risk of tobacco-related cancers in a cohort of French women. *Journal of the National Cancer Institute* 97(18): 1338–44. Virtamo, J., et al. 2003. Incidence of cancer and mortality following alpha-tocopherol and beta-carotene supplementation: A postintervention follow-up. *Journal of the American Medical Association* 290(4): 476–85.

8. Gaziano, J. M. 2004. Vitamin E and cardiovascular disease: Observational studies. *Annals of the New York Academy of Science* 1031: 280–91. McQueen, M. J., et al. 2005. The HOPE (Heart Outcomes Prevention Evaluation) Study and its consequences. *Scandinavian Journal of Clinical and Laboratory Investigation* 240: 143–56.

9. Yoshida, M., et al. 2004. Dietary indole-3-carbinol promotes endometrial adeno-carcinoma development in rats initiated with N-ethyl-N'-nitro-N-nitroso-guanidine, with induction of cytochrome P450s in the liver and consequent modulation of estrogen metabolism. *Carcinogenesis* 25(11): 2257–64.

10. Moon, Y. J., X. Wang, and M. E. Morris. 2005. Dietary flavonoids: Effects on xenobiotic and carcinogen metabolism. *Toxicology In Vitro* 20(2): 187–210. Review. Hodek, P., P. Trefil, and M. Stiborova. 2002. Flavonoids-potent and versatile biologically active compounds interacting with cytochromes P450. *Chemical and Biological Interactions* 139(1): 1–21.

11. Mazza, G., et al. 2002. Absorption of anthocyanins from blueberries and serum antioxidant status in human subjects. *Journal of Agricultural and Food Chemistry* 50(26): 7731–37.

12. Morand, C., et al. 1998. Plasma metabolites of quercetin and their antioxidant properties. *American Journal of Physiology* 275(1 pt 2): R212–19. de Groot, H., and U. Rauen. 1998. Tissue injury by reactive oxygen species and the protective effects of flavonoids. *Fundamentals of Clinical Pharmacology* 12(3): 249–55.

13. Cody, V., E. Middleton, and J. B. Harborne. 1988. *Plant Flavonoids in Biology and Medicine II.* Alan R. Liss, Inc. 135–38.

14. Hruby, K., et al. 1983. Chemotherapy of *Amanita phalloides* poisoning with intravenous silibinin. *Human Toxicology* 2: 183–95. Salmi, H. A., and S. Sarna. 1982. Effect of silymarin on chemical, functional, and morphological alterations of the liver. A double-blind controlled study. *Scandinavian Journal of Gastroenterology* 17(4): 517–21. Wu, C. G., et al. 1993. Protective effect of silymarin on rat liver injury induced by isdhemia. *Virchows Archiv B: Cell Pathology Including Molecular Pathology* 64: 259–63. Pietrangelo, A., et al. 1995. Antioxidant activity of silybin in vivo during long-term iron overload in rats. *Gastroenterology* 109: 1941–49. Kropacova, K., E. Misurova, and H. Hakova. 1998. Protective and therapeutic effect of silymarin on the development of latent liver damage. *Radiatsionnaia biologiia, radioecologiia* 38: 411–15. Campos R., et al. 1989. Silybin dihemisuccinate protects against glutathione depletion and lipid peroxidation induced by acetaminophen on rat liver. *Planta Medica* 55: 417–19.

15. Dwivedi, C., et al. 1990. Effect of calcium glucarate on beta-glucuronidase activity and glucarate content of certain vegetables and fruits. *Biochemical Medicine and Metabolic Biology* 43(2): 83–92. Nijhoff, W. A., et al. 1995. Effects of consumption of Brussels sprouts on plasma and urinary glutathione S-transferase class-alpha and -pi in humans. *Carcinogenesis* 16(4): 955–57.

16. Khashab, M., A. J. Tector, and P. Y. Kwo. 2007. Epidemiology of acute liver failure. *Current Gastroenterology Reports* 9(1): 66–73.

17. Biewenga, G., et al. 1997. The pharmacology of the antioxidant lipoic acid. *General Pharmacology* 29: 315–31. Khanna, S., et al. 1999. Alpha-lipoic acid supplementation: Tissue glutathione homeostasis at rest and after exercise. *Journal of Applied Physiology* 86(4): 1191–96. Han, D., et al. 1997. Lipoic acid increases de novo synthesis of cellular glutathione by improving cysteine utilization. *Biofactors* 6(3): 321–8. Bustamante, J., et al. 1998. Alpha-lipoic acid in liver metabolism and disease. *Free Radical Biology and Medicine* 24(6): 1023–39.

Chapter 2

1. Hourigan, C. S. 2006. The molecular basis of celiac disease. *Clinical and Experimental Medicine* 6(2): 53–59.

2. Sandiford, C. P., et al. 1997. Identification of the major water/salt insoluble wheat proteins involved in cereal hypersensitivity. *Clinical and Experimental Allergy* 27: 1120–29.

3. Stoersrud, S., et al. 2003. Adult coeliac disease patients do tolerate large amounts of oats. *European Journal of Clinical Nutrition* 57: 163–69. Hoegberg, L., et al. 2004. Oats to children with newly diagnosed coeliac disease: A randomised double blind study. *Gut* 54: 645–54.

4. Torres, M. I., M. A. Lopez Casado, and A. Rios. 2007. New aspects in celiac disease. *World Journal of Gastroenterology* 13(8): 1156–61.

5. Shattock, P. and P. Whiteley. 2002. Biochemical aspects in autism spectrum disorders: updating the opioid-excess theory and presenting new opportunities for biomedical intervention. *Expert Opinion on Therapeutic Targets.* 6: 175-183. See ESPA Research for more details (www.espa-research.org.uk).

6. Fukudome, S., Y. Jinsmaa, T. Matsukawa, R. Sasaki, and M. Yoshikawa. 1997. Release of opioid peptides, gluten exorphins by the action of pancreatic elastase. *Federation of European Biochemical Sciences Letters.* 412: 475-479.

7. U.S. National Institutes of Health (http://digestive.niddk.nih .gov/ddiseases/pubs/lactoseintolerance/).

8. LeRoith, D., and C. T. Roberts, Jr. 2003. The insulin-like growth factor system and cancer. *Cancer Letters* 195(2): 127–37. Review.

9. Juliano, L. M., and R. R. Griffiths. 2004. A critical review of caffeine withdrawal: Empirical validation of symptoms and signs, incidence, severity, and associated features. *Psychopharmacology* 176(1): 1–29.

10. Rogers, P. J., et al. 2005. Effects of caffeine and caffeine withdrawal on mood and cognitive performance degraded by sleep restriction. *Psychopharmacology* 179(4): 742–52.

11. Gilliland, K., and D. Adress. 1981. Ad lib caffeine consumption, symptoms of caffeinism, and academic performance. *American Journal of Psychiatry* 138(4): 512–14.

12. Institute for Optimum Nutrition, 100% Health Survey 2010, Holford & Associates. See www.patrickholford.com.

13. Vlachopoulos, C., et al. 2005. Chronic coffee consumption has a detrimental effect on aortic stiffness and wave reflections. *American Journal of Clinical Nutrition* 81(6): 1307–12.

14. Refsum, H., et al. 2006. The Hordaland Homocysteine Study: A community-based study of homocysteine, its determinants, and associations with disease. *Journal of Nutrition* 136: 1731S–40S.

15. Zampelas, A., et al. 2004. Associations between coffee consumption and inflammatory markers in healthy persons: The ATTICA study. *American Journal of Clinical Nutrition* 80(4): 862–67.

16. Shilo, L., et al. 2002. The effects of coffee consumption on sleep and melatonin secretion. *Sleep Medicine* 3(3): 271–73.

17. Waluga, M., and M. Hartleb. 2003. Alcoholic liver disease. *Wiadomosci Lekarskie* 56(1–2): 61–70. Review. Bae, K. S., et al. 2004. The short term prognosis in alcoholic liver disease with metabolic acidosis. *Korean Journal of Hepatology* 10(2): 117–24.

18. World Cancer Research Fund and American Institute for Cancer Research. 1997. *Food, Nutrition and the Prevention of Cancer: A Global Perspective*. American Institute for Cancer Research. Chapter 5.5.

Chapter 3

1. Thomas. B., ed. 2001. *Manual of Dietetic Practice*, 3rd ed. Blackwell Publishing.

2. Kleiner, S. M. 1999. Water: An essential but overlooked nutrient. *Journal of the American Dietetic Association* 99(2): 200–6.

3. Thomas. B., ed. 2001. *Manual of Dietetic Practice*, 3rd ed. Blackwell Publishing.

4. Batmanghelidj, F. 1992. *Your Body's Many Cries for Water*. Global Health Solutions.

5. Durga, J., et al. 2007. Effect of a 3-year folic acid supplementation on cognitive function in older adults in the FACIT trial: A randomised, double blind, controlled trial. *Lancet* 369 (9557): 208–16.

6. Block, G. 1991. Epidemiologic evidence regarding vitamin C and cancer. *American Journal of Clinical Nutrition* 54(6 Suppl): 1310S–14S.

7. Nijhoff, W., et al. 1995. Effects of consumption of Brussels sprouts on intestinal and lymphocytic glutathione S-transferases in humans. *Carcinogenesis* 16(9): 2125–28.

Resources

Food allergies or sensitivities

Immuno Laboratories offers a home test kit for food allergy (IgG ELISA) and homocysteine testing. With this you can take your own pinprick blood sample and return it to the lab for analysis. This test identifies if you have any food allergies to any of 88, 115, or 154 foods (depending on which assay you choose), including gluten and gliadin. Food allergy testing is best done under the guidance of a nutritional therapist.

Contact Immuno Laboratories at (800) 231-9197 or visit www.immunolabs.com.

Nutrition Consultations

One-on-one nutrition consultations are available through naturopathic physicians, nutritionists, and physicians trained in the optimum nutrition approach. The following organizations can help you find a practitioner in your area.

American Association for Health Freedom
4620 Lee Highway, Suite 210
Arlington, VA 22207
(800) 230 2762
www.apma.net

American Association of Naturopathic Physicians
4435 Wisconsin Avenue NW
Suite 403
Washington, DC 20016
(866) 538-2267
www.naturopathic.org

American College for advancement in Medicine

24411 Ridge Route
Suite 115
Laguna Hills, CA 92653
(888) 439-6891
www.acam.org

American Holistic Medical Association

1 Eagle Valley Court
Suite 201
Broadview Heights, OH 44147
(440) 838-1010
www.holisticmedicine.org

Metagenics

100 Ave La Pata
San Clemente, CA 92673
(800) 962-9400
www.metagenics.com

Patrick Holford organizations

The Holford Diet Club

provides advice and support
for weight loss, including
many of the detox principles.
For more information, visit
www.holforddiet.com.

The Institute for Optimum Nutrition (ION) maintains a

list of nutrition practitioners,
an information service, and
a quarterly journal, *Optimum*
Nutrition. For more information, visit www.ion.ac.uk.

Psychocalisthenics

Psychocalisthenics is an exercise system that takes less than
twenty minutes a day, devel-
ops strength, suppleness, and
stamina, and generates vital
energy. See the book *Master
Level Exercise: Psychocalisthenics*
and the Psychocalisthenics CD
and DVD. For further information, see www.pcals.com.

Supplements

Enzymatic Therapy

The website has a "where to
buy" function for retail stores
and online e-stores.
(800) 783-2286
www.enzy.com

Nature's Plus

The website has a store locator.
www.naturesplus.com

Solgar Vitamin and Herb

The website has a "where to
buy" function for retail stores
and online e-stores.
(877) 765-4274
(877-SOLGAR-4)
www.solgar.com

Source Naturals

The website has a "where to buy" function for retail stores and online e-stores.
(800) 815-2333
www.sourcenaturals.com

Twinlab Corporation

The website gives product information only.
(800) 645-5626
www.twinlab.com

Tests

Laboratory tests are available for all the tests mentioned in this book, through nutritionists. Leading laboratories include the following.

Genova Diagnostics

Offers Liver Detoxification Capacity Profile. This urine test identifies how effective your body's phase I and Phase II detoxification is. This helps identify which nutrients are important to include in your detox diet, and which substances are especially important for you to avoid.
63 Zillicoa Street
Asheville, NC 28801-1074
(800) 522-4762
www.genovadiagnostics.com

Immuno Laboratories

Offers IgE and IgG food allergy testing.
6801 Powerline Road
Fort Lauderdale, FL 33309
(800) 231-9197
www.immunolabs.com

Vitamin Diagnostics

Offers a urinary HPL test.
Route 35, Industrial Drive
Cliffwood Beach, NJ 07735
(732) 583-7773

York Nutritional Laboratories

Offers a wide range of tests and specializes in testing that utilizes finger-prick blood samples that can be carried out at home. Includes the IgG ELISA (food intolerance) test.
(888) 751-3388
www.yorkallergyusa.com

Recommended Reading List

Baker, Sidney M. 2003. *Detoxification and Healing.* McGraw-Hill.

Bland, Jeffrey. 1997. *The 20-Day Rejuvenation Diet Program.* Keats Publishing.

Holford, Patrick. 2005. *The New Optimum Nutrition Bible.* The Crossing Press.

———. 2004. *The Holford Low-GL Diet.* Piatkus Books.

——— and Fiona McDonald Joyce. 2005. *The Holford Low-GL Diet Cookbook.* Piatkus Books.

———. 1999. *Improve Your Digestion.* Piatkus Books.

Lipski, Elizabeth. 1996. *Digestive Wellness.* Keats Publishing.

Index

Printed in the United States
by Baker & Taylor Publisher Services